Other books by the author

Sports Injuries: A Self-Help Guide
Knee Health: Problems, Prevention and Cure
Strokes and Head Injuries: A Guide for Patients, Families
    Friends and Carers (with Mary Lynch)
Children and Sport: Fitness, Injuries and Diet
Running: Fitness and Injuries – A Self-Help Guide

THE BACK

PROBLEMS AND PREVENTION

A Self-Help Guide

Vivian Grisogono

JOHN MURRAY
Albemarle Street, London

First published in 1996
by John Murray (Publishers) Ltd.,
50 Albemarle Street, London W1X 4BD

A catalogue record for this book is available from the British Library

Readers are advised to seek professional help in any case of
injury. The author and publishers cannot be held responsible
for readers' injuries in any circumstances.

ISBN 0–7195–5531 0

Typeset in Sabon and Gill

Printed and bound in Great Britain by Butler and Tanner Limited, Frome
and London.

For Lydia

Contents

Acknowledgements   viii

Introduction   ix

1. Sports, activities and dangers to the back and neck   1

2. Everyday life and your back and neck   15

3. Structure and functions of the back and neck   39

4. Pain in the back and neck   63

5. Coping with back and neck pain   85

6. Practitioners and treatment methods   93

7. Spinal conditions and diagnosis   121

8. Exercise tests   153

9. Remedial exercises for the back, neck and related joints   179

10. Health, fitness training and your back   199

Recommended reading   219

Index   224

Acknowledgements

I sincerely thank the following people for helping me in various ways during the preparation of this book: Martin Creasey, Churchill Livingstone Publishers, Trinda Dover, Jovan and Ljiljana Djurovic, John Fitzgerald and 'Snappy Snaps', Chiswick, Richard and Tasya Gardner, Roger Hudson, Johan Jeronimus, Grant McIntyre, John Murray, Flora Pedler and her colleagues from the Society of Orthopaedic Medicine Council, Chris and Lizzie Phillips, Stuart Phillips, Gerry Quaghebeur, Lisa Quine and The Back Store, Peter Richards, David Walters, Debra Wilkinson, Floyd Williams, and Houghtons Book Suppliers.

Special thanks go to those who have provided the book with visual imagery: to Michael Bartlett, as always, for his diagrams and delightful cartoons; Peter Gardiner for his expert anatomical drawings and diagrams; and to Richard Gardner for his special photographs.

Very special gratitude is due to Gail Pirkis for the patience, efficiency and skill with which she enacted her starring role in persuading this book into shape and out (almost) on time.

Introduction

It was because I had a bad back at a young age that I became a chartered physiotherapist, a career move I have never regretted. For four years it had seemed that no one could help me, until Mr E. Sohikish, a chartered physiotherapist specializing in injured tennis players, set me on the rehabilitation programme that has kept my back healthy from that time to this. To him I remain eternally grateful. What I suffered and learned then, and what I know now, have been the inspirations for this book.

Spinal problems are so common that hardly anyone escapes back or neck pain. It may happen early on in one's life or in later years. However strong you are, there is no guarantee that back or neck pain will never happen to you, just because you may have escaped it so far.

Working days lost through spinal pain cost every industrialized country huge sums each year. For the individual there may be financial loss, but the cost is also calculated in terms of physical distress, emotional upset and loss of pleasurable leisure pursuits. Children's spinal problems give particular cause for concern: they may be serious in themselves, or they may have harmful long-term consequences.

This book sets out the risks of back or neck injuries which exist in sports, workplaces, and daily activities of all kinds. By explaining how the spine works and what its limitations are, it aims to spell out how to avoid some kinds of back or neck problems, and what to do in certain situations of pain. Spinal problems can be complex, and self-help for back and neck problems is strictly limited. It is vital to understand what kind of help you should look for, and how to make the best of the professional expertise available.

Above all, this is a book about healthy and safe exercising. The right kind of exercise at the right time combined with a positive approach can help physical recovery from most of the common spinal problems.

Vivian Grisogono
January 1996

Sports, activities and dangers to the back and neck

1

The backbone is the vital central area of the human body, linking the pelvis to the ribs, shoulder girdle and head. It is more technically known as the vertebral column, spinal column or spine (although sometimes people use the term spine to mean the spinal cord, which is part of the central nervous system and not part of the bone structure). The structure and functions of the back and neck are complicated, and so they have an apparently limitless capacity for injury, damage and causing pain. It is not surprising that 'back problems' are among the most common complaints treated by doctors and therapists of all kinds. It is generally agreed that the majority of people probably suffer back pain at one time or another during their lives.

As everywhere in the human body, the structure of the back and neck is closely related to their functions. It is because the back has to perform a variety of different functions, some of which are not necessarily easily compatible, that the structure of the back is so complex and its capacity for injury is so great.

POSTURAL CONTROL AND MUSCLE TONE

The human body functions in relation to the force of gravity, so that even when we are 'doing nothing' some muscles may have to be active to maintain a postural position. Our joints, ligaments and muscles are geared to holding the body upright against gravity when we are standing, sitting or kneeling, and to providing stability when we want to activate

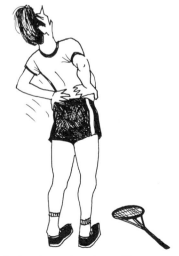

Back pain can be a hazard in many sports

muscles to create joint movements. In general, the muscles which control posture are deep-seated, close to the body's bone framework, and they contain a predominance of red slow-twitch muscle fibres, which allows them to contract repetitively without getting tired quickly. Muscle tone is the state of tension in any muscle. With normal tone, the muscle is ready to contract according to need.

Normal tone in fact varies according to the individual. Most active athletes have generally higher tone muscles than inactive people. If muscle tone is abnormally high, the muscles are tight, and may be difficult to contract at will, because they are already in a state of contraction (technically in spasm). When muscle tone is low, it is hard to activate them, as they are not really prepared for action. Normal muscles can become low in tone through depression or a low mood, or after a long period of bed-rest for illness or injury.

Gravity provides a strong downward pressure on the body. When lying down, the body is fully supported against this load. Because of this, most people are about $\frac{3}{4}$ inch (2cm) longer lying down than standing up. We tend to 'shrink' very slightly during the day, especially in the first hour after getting up in the morning. The amount of shrinkage is a little greater after standing for a long period than after sitting, and most noticeable after carrying heavy weights. With increasing age, there is a steady decrease in the overall length of the backbone, but as this happens, the daily variation gets less.

The normal curves of the spine develop in relation to gravity. The forward curve of the neck (cervical lordosis) develops when a baby is about three months old and starts to lift its head up against gravity while lying on its stomach. The forward curve in the lower back (lumbar lordosis) forms as the baby begins to extend its legs and take weight through them, usually somewhere between the first year and eighteen months. In females, the lumbar lordosis becomes more pronounced during the childbearing years, probably under hormonal influences, and it tends to be slightly flatter before the onset of periods (menarche) and after the menopause. Wearing shoes with very high heels also increases the lumbar curve, because the trunk has to tip forwards slightly to balance the body and keep it upright. This can be especially harmful during the the critical development period of the teenage years.

In between the curves of the low back and the neck, the upper back slopes the other way, backwards (technically into

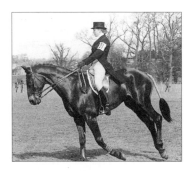

Sitting upright for dressage: the lower the knees, the straighter the back, and the more pronounced the low-back curve

a thoracic kyphosis). The degree of each curve varies according to the individual, partly through hereditary and congenital factors, partly through postural habits and physical activities, and partly through the effects of the growth and ageing processes. In old age, especially among females, the thoracic curve can become very hunched, and this is known as a 'dowager's hump'.

Some people have very pronounced curves, others flatter, straighter spines. Many people have a degree of sideways twisting and bending, called a scoliosis. This can happen for a variety of reasons, and is not a problem if it is only slight. A minor degree of scoliosis can happen through intensive sports activities involving twisting and bending the spine, especially if the player is a teenager, and the sport involves moving predominantly in a repetitive arc of movement, as in rowing or using the dominant arm while bending and twisting the trunk, for instance in tennis.

Injuries can affect the curvature of the spine. There may be muscle tightness (technically spasm) on one side of the vertebral column which pulls the joints sideways and creates a temporary scoliosis, with or without pain. Using crutches for a leg injury, or limping for a long time can also cause a sideways pull on the spine, which can remain an habitual pattern, even after the leg has recovered full function. Injury in the groin region usually causes a reflex bending (flexion) in the hip. This is a protective mechanism, but unfortunately it can cause a compensatory arching in the lower back, forcibly increasing the lumbar lordosis, and so risking strain on the lumbar joints.

Theoretically, the line of gravity passes vertically downwards through the body when one is upright. Where the line passes directly through a bone or joint, it places a special load on that point; when it lies in front, behind or beside a bone or joint, the loading is exerted so that the muscles lying on the opposite side have to work harder if they are to prevent the body from falling into the direction of gravity's pull.

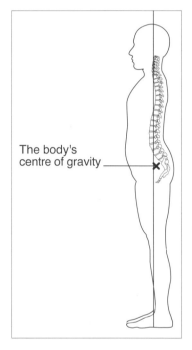

The body's centre of gravity

The line of gravity and centre of gravity in relation to the upright body

BODY BALANCE

The normal human body develops functionally according to in-built capacities and according to need. Habitual posture and physical activities play key roles in dictating how our bodies develop and change from earliest childhood to old

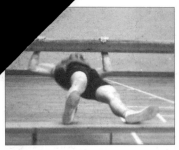

A one-sided sport like rowing creates body imbalance, making it difficult to do a symmetrical exercise like lying-down pull-ups correctly

age. Within the basic format of the normal human body, there are apparently endless individual variations, some of which we are born with, others which we acquire through circumstances.

Some of the structural influences on the spinal joints

- Handedness
- Pelvic tilt: front-back (antero-posterior), sideways (lateral)
- Leg length differences: true or apparent shortening
- Stiff hip(s) and hip joint discrepancies
- Leg alignment
- Foot alignment and malfunction
- Tight or weak back extensor muscles
- Tight or weak abdominal muscles
- Tight or weak hip abductor muscles
- Tight or weak gluteal muscles
- Tight or weak pectoral muscles
- Stiff shoulders
- Malfunction in the joints of the shoulder girdle

The human body is designed more or less symmetrically, in that to either side of the central trunk formation we have limbs which are constructed with the same bone, joint and muscle structures on each side. However, there may be structural discrepancies from birth, and many more are likely to develop through the growth and ageing processes.

One of the primary causes of asymmetrical development is 'handedness'. If your dominant hand is *very* dominant and you are very one-sided, you can create over-development in the muscles of one side of the body relative to the other. Gradually, this can contribute to limitation of joint movement, which in later years can be linked to degeneration in the joints. Racket games, for instance, can lead to these developments, especially if the player started very young (pre-teen) and played intensively through the teenage growth period. Fencing is a sport which can create very pronounced body asymmetry, with over-development of the dominant arm and leg, rotational distortion of the spinal joints, and relative under-development of the non-dominant side.

In human beings, the arms are relatively less strong than the legs, so there is normally a discrepancy between the upper and lower halves of the body. If this imbalance increases because you use your legs much more than your arms in your daily activities, your neck and upper back may lose much of their normal muscle protection. This can happen if you do a lot of walking, running or football (soccer).

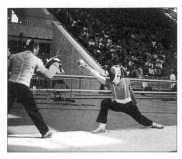

Fencing creates severe distorting stresses on the spine

There is probably no such thing as the 'perfect' body, and no clear-cut rules about the best or worst types of body structure. What we ask of our bodies is that they should operate efficiently for the tasks we want or need to perform, without limitation or pain. For good overall physical movement patterns, all the body's interrelating joints and muscles need to co-ordinate smoothly.

Joint limitations inevitably interfere with efficient body mechanics. For instance, if your hips are stiff, movements involving them may create extra, abnormal pressures through the sacroiliac joints into the low back. Stiff hips may be something you were born with. Sometimes hip stiffness can be due to poor foot function, especially if you tend to over-pronate, so that your feet fold inwards when you walk and run. Stiff shoulders can also cause increased pressure on the low back if you try to do activities requiring full stretch in the shoulders. If there is joint limitation on one side of the body and not the other, the alteration in body mechanics is even more dangerous because it causes asymmetrical stresses across the body and especially through the spinal joints.

Many people have differences in their leg lengths, and in some cases this asymmetry contributes to back pain because it causes an awkward tilting of the pelvis when you stand, walk or run. There are in fact two types of leg length discrepancy: 'real shortening', in which the bones of one leg can be measured as being shorter than the other, and 'apparent shortening', where the legs seem to be different lengths because the pelvis or low back has tilted sideways, pulling one leg upwards and compressing the other side.

Because of our functional needs, some muscles in the body are relatively stronger than others: for instance, the quadriceps muscles are normally stronger than the hamstrings in the leg, and the biceps stronger than the triceps in the arm. It is also the case that some muscle groups may be relatively tighter than others. This can be due to your individual structure, or to phases in your body development. The effect is often especially marked during the teenage growth phases, when increased bone length can make the hamstrings particularly tight. A similar effect can happen through ageing, if joints such as the hips deteriorate and lose their full range of movement.

The development of significant muscle imbalance inevitably has a bad effect on co-ordinated biomechanical actions. The need to compensate for weakness or tightness in one area automatically throws extra pressure on to another. The correct position of the pelvis can only be maintained if all the muscles which support it are consistent in their strength and length. Weakness in one area or another of the trunk itself can throw increased stress on to the spinal joints, especially weakness in the abdominal muscles, perhaps following childbirth or abdominal surgery, or through plain lack of condition. Back problems cause muscular inefficiency in the affected area. There may be muscle strain or rupture, in which case the injured muscle cannot function properly until it has healed and regained its full elasticity. Any kind of spinal joint problem usually gives rise to a protective muscle spasm, or tightening, around the painful joint, and this too prevents the muscle from working normally.

Muscle imbalance anywhere in the body can have a harmful effect on the spinal muscles and joints. Compensation is the inevitable result of injuries. If you limp because of a foot or leg injury, you distort the normal actions of the hips and pelvis, which in turn causes rotational stresses in the lower back. For a long-standing shoulder injury, such as a dislocation or fracture, the arm is usually immobilized in a harness or sling which keeps the arm close to the body. If your arm is immobilized in a sling, you overuse the other side, and create unbalanced stresses through the shoulder girdle and middle back. This is why it is so important to try to avoid immobilizing any part of the body following injury if it is at all possible to keep it moving. Any enforced period of rest should be kept to the minimum possible.

It is absolutely essential to do rehabilitation exercises to restore full normal movement after *any* injury which has resulted in immobilization (or relative rest) before you return to full sporting activities. It is dangerous to assume that you will recover full function naturally without special re-training focused on the injured area. The chances are that you will be left with a deficit which, however slight, will create body imbalance together with the risk of secondary injury.

Sometimes body imbalance leading to abnormal stresses on the spine is caused by over-zealous prophylactic protection of other joints. I remember a painfully dramatic incident at a major international competition, when a male gymnast, with both ankles heavily taped to protect against ankle sprain, landed gracefully and symmetrically from the high bar. However, as his ankles were rigidly encased in taping, they could not bend and give normally and so remained stiff. This in turn prevented the gymnast's knees and hips from bending and yielding to take up the compression forces. As he landed, there was a loud crack: something in his lower back had given, he fell to the floor, and was stretchered off. It was a sad and salutary reminder of how much the body-weight is multiplied when someone jumps down from a great height, and how important it is for all the interrelated joints to be able to function freely and fully in order to dissipate compression forces.

FUNCTION AND HARM

When it moves, the spine is subject to a great number of complex forces. Compression forces jar or push the joints, traction forces pull the joints apart, shearing forces stretch the joints obliquely at awkward angles, and rotational stresses occur through twisting movements. Most actions involve a combination of these forces. In general, the arrangement of the spinal joints and their supporting structures, the ligaments, discs and muscles, is adequate to absorb the forces and therefore prevent injury. However, if the forces are greater than the ability of the joints and muscles to withstand them, something has to give, and damage can result.

Spinal damage caused by a sudden bad accident such as a car smash, a parachute failing to open, or diving into shallow water, is logical and understandable. What often surprises people is how easily acute back problems can happen: sometimes they seem to happen without any rhyme or reason at all. A common story is that of someone simply bending over, perhaps brushing his or her teeth or pulling on socks or tights; there is a sudden sharp 'bang' or stab of pain in the lower back and then it is very hard to straighten up again. The mechanism of this type of injury is much harder to understand, as it seems to come on 'out of the blue'. In fact, there is usually a reason for it, even if the reason is sometimes very obscure and hard to identify.

Risk factors in spinal injuries

Injury to the back or neck is more likely to happen if:
- a sudden major force is applied to the spine
- the spine is going through a growth and development phase (especially in the late teens)
- the spinal joints and structures have degenerated through ageing (wear and tear), disease or previous injury
- the musculature supporting the spine is relatively weak, tight or unbalanced
- the biomechanical function of the spine is inefficient due to fatigue, hormone influences, illness or injury
- related joints which should assimilate some of the forces on the spine are not functioning properly
- the movement patterns you are performing are unfamiliar, difficult, limited or repetitive
- equipment or opponents are not size-matched to the person
- the environment is not appropriate to the activity

RISKS TO THE BACK AND NECK THROUGH SPORTS

Most sports inevitably stress the spine in one way or another. Anyone involved in sport, whether as participant, coach, instructor or physical education teacher, should be aware of the special risks attached to different types of physical activity. It is also essential to be trained in first-aid, so that you can act promptly and correctly, should an accident occur. Awareness of how injuries can happen is, of course, important for knowing how to minimize or prevent the risks.

Some sports carry the risk of violent overload on the spine, especially if they involve potential contact, collisions and falls, as in rugby, American football, ice hockey, horse riding, show jumping, wrestling, skiing, ski-jumping and parachuting. Breaking the spinal cord through trauma is the biggest

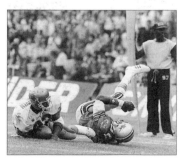

American football can involve heavy falls

danger in this type of sport. Once the spinal cord is completely disrupted, it cannot repair itself, as the central nervous system has no capacity for regeneration, so the victim is likely to be completely paralysed below the level of the break. However, functional recovery is possible if the spinal cord is not completely ruptured.

Most sports cause compression, shearing or traction stresses on the spinal joints. One of these forces may predominate, but more often the spinal stresses occur in combination. Many sports cause repetitive stresses which can create body imbalance and cumulatively lead to overload of the spinal bones, muscles and joint structures. Only a few sports, such as karate and gymnastics, consist of movement patterns which are sufficiently varied and comprehensive to provide all-round body conditioning and therefore good body balance.

Compression forces on the back and neck can be the result of sports such as heavy weightlifting or powerlifting, horse riding and show jumping, acrobatics, parachuting, stunt flying, or racing in fast cars or speedboats. The compressive effects may be from sudden massive loading of the spine through lifting a heavy weight or through impact. They are often cumulative, either because the movements are repeated frequently, as in powerlifting or show jumping, or because the sport involves periods of continual repetitive pressure, such as the buffeting in fast motorboats, or the 'g' forces created in Formula One racing cars and aeroplanes used for acrobatics.

Trampolining, diving and the Fosbury Flop high jump technique are activities which demand fast and precise trunk movements in the air, causing shearing, twisting stresses on the spine. Landing, especially from the Fosbury Flop, can cause problems through jarring and compression, either through cumulative strain due to repetitive practice, or through the sudden extra trauma of an awkward landing. The triple jump is a complicated discipline technically, requiring excellent leg strength, balance and co-ordination to withstand the compressive pressure of landing and pushing off hard from each foot.

Female gymnasts need maximum flexibility in all joints, including the spine, besides sufficient strength to move their bodyweight around at speed. A gymnast's natural build influences her technique: for instance, the gymnast whose shoulders are naturally relatively stiff has to compensate by

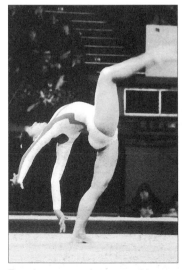

Female gymnasts have to cultivate extreme flexibility in the spine

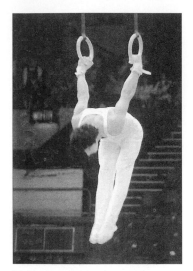

Male gymnasts need strength through the whole body

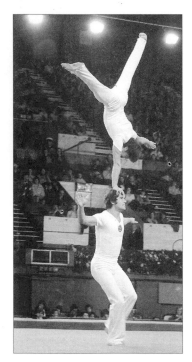

Compression exerted through the gymnast's neck and spine by the effect of gravity and the partner's full bodyweight

increasing the arch of her back (lordosis) in order to stretch her arms fully up above her head. Any slight stiffness in the hips forces the lower back to arch more when the gymnast does straight or sideways 'splits'. Being very flexible naturally is not necessarily an advantage, if the gymnast's joint stability is insufficient to match and control the range of movement. Forcing excessive joint movement, especially in unusual ranges such as full spinal backwards bending (hyperextension) can lead to problems later on when the bones are fully developed.

Tumbling and vaulting can involve full bending, extending, twisting and shearing movements in the air. There are then large compression forces through the spine when the gymnast lands on her feet or hands, as the weight of the gymnast's body is effectively multiplied because of her speed and the height from which she reaches the ground. Gymnastic mats provide cushioning when the gymnast lands from the vaulting horse, beam or asymmetric bars. However, floor routines are done on a resilient surface, usually barefoot or in wafer-thin pumps, so there is little shock absorption. And all this pressure has to be absorbed by an immature skeleton!

In male gymnastics, the disciplines are geared to a combination of strength and speed which can only be achieved successfully once the body is fairly mature. The direct and cumulative pressures on the spine can be very great, if not enormous, and they are of course multiplied in the events where two or more gymnasts work together in loading and supporting roles.

Tennis probably produces more and worse back injuries than other racket sports. It requires a lot of twisting movement through the spine, together with a complex combination of bending and extending, as a stroke may have to be played overhead, from the feet, at waist height or at shoulder level. The two-handed player may over-stress the thoracic spine (upper back), whereas a hard-hitting one-handed player is more vulnerable to sacroiliac and lumbar spine (lower back) strains.

Although the back can be injured by an awkward stroke in players of any standard, serious or professional tennis players are most at risk of bad back problems. Apart from the repetitive twisting strain of continual stroke production, the sport can involve quite heavy loading, especially in the men's power game on grass or any other fast surface. Playing a lot of tennis from an early age inevitably causes muscular imbalance through the whole trunk from shoulders to pelvis, and this can create a mild scoliosis, which in turn can make the player more prone to episodes of back pain.

The forces exerted through a tennis player's body vary according to whether the game is played on a forgiving surface like clay or an unyielding surface like cement; whether the racket is heavy or light, head-heavy or not, thick or thin-gripped, and tightly or loosely strung; the quality of the player's timing, and the incidence of mis-hits; whether the player is powerful and hits through each stroke at high speed, or plays more defensively; whether he or she is a volleying net player or a ground-stroke baseline retriever; whether the style is mainly top-spin, under-spin or 'flat' style; if the serve is 'cannonball', top-spin or any other style, including under-arm; how the opponent plays; and how often the player practises and plays matches.

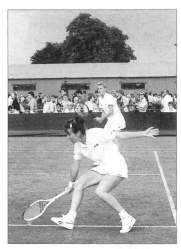

Twisting movements at speed can cause back problems in tennis players

By contrast with tennis and badminton, squash involves a lot of bending and twisting trunk movements at high speed, without much movement stretching upwards, in the British version of the game played on heated courts. The constant crouching and lunging movements place particular stresses on the knees, hips and lower back. Most players use one hand on the racket, resulting in shearing stresses felt especially over one or both sacroiliac joints. For the rare two-handed squash player, there may be relatively more shearing stress in the thoracic spine (upper back) than lower down, as lunging reach is limited and the ball has to be struck from closer to the body. Golf, like squash, involves bending and twisting to strike the ball with the club. However, golf is even more stressful for the spinal joints than squash, because the precise rotational movements required for each full golf stroke take the body through a very difficult arc of movement involving the hips, pelvis, spine and shoulder girdle. As there are no backhands in golf, repetitive practice is restricted to a smaller range of movements than in squash, therefore creating an even greater risk of body imbalance.

All sports which involve batting and bowling, including cricket and baseball, can have stressful effects on the spine, not only for the person striking with the bat, but also for the bowler or pitcher. At the speed with which each ball is delivered, the spine is taken through severe shearing stresses each time. These can very quickly go beyond safe limits if the player does long periods of repetitive practice. Throwing events such as the javelin, hammer and shot use different delivery techniques, but carry similar risks to bowling and pitching, because they all involve explosive rotational stresses which are often practised repetitively. Wheelchair athletes who practise sports involving repetitive explosive effort, such as the throws and archery, should also be aware of the dangers of developing harmful body imbalance through repetitive practice.

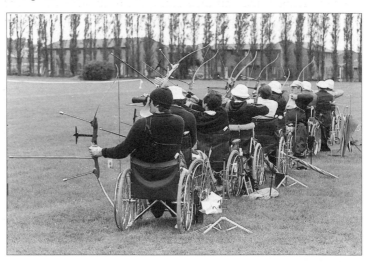

Wheelchair athletes in sports like archery must also do exercises to prevent body imbalance

Just as throwing puts pressure on the spinal joints from the effort exerted by the shoulder girdle, kicking a ball hard, as in football (soccer), rugby or American football, can cause shearing through over-stress of the hips and pelvic joints. The result can be disruption of the pelvic joints, especially the pubic and sacroiliac joints, possibly combined with damage in the low back. The effect is worse if the player is very one-sided and always kicks with the dominant foot, as this can create cumulative joint imbalance around the hips and pelvis, which is of course a dangerous background for sports involving explosive, potentially traumatic forces.

Cycling and running are repetitive-movement sports which use mainly leg strength. If they are used for fitness training, they strengthen the legs, but do little for the trunk, shoulders and arms. Canoeing, by contrast, uses the upper body, but does little for the legs. The more cycling and running you do, the greater the imbalance between the fitness of your legs and the relative lack of fitness of your upper body. The converse can be said for canoeing. In either case, there is a need to redress the balance through appropriate training. For the runner, the imbalance not only increases the risk of back problems, but also reduces running efficiency, as your arms are needed for propulsion, and if they tire easily through lack of training, they will be a limiting factor on any long run.

Running can cause jarring stresses into the pelvis and low back from repetitive pounding, especially if you run long distances on hard surfaces. Running on camber or around bends on the racing track can also cause shearing stresses on the pelvis and low back, combined with compressive pressure on the hip. Cycling does not cause jarring stresses, but it can cause a potentially damaging sideways tilt of the pelvis if the saddle is even slightly too high. On a racing bike, the rider's

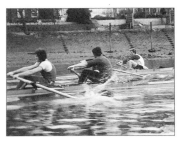
Rowers need strong backs

Possible risks to the spine through sports

Potentially harmful effects of sports on the body:
- Joint distortion
- Bone stress
- Muscle imbalance

Injury causes:
- Shearing stresses
- Jarring stresses
- Over-stretch
- Overload

Injuries:
- Acute traumatic injuries
- Cumulative overuse strains
- Strains due to poor body mechanics

hunched position can cause a flattening of the normal curve of the low back, leading to loss of the normal movement range in the spinal joints. Racing cyclists often have surprisingly straight backs when they stand up: this is because they have to lift their head up to see forwards on the bike, and the extension of the neck compensates for the hunched position of the low back.

Rowers, by contrast, tend to have very hunched shoulders when they stand up, because modern rowing technique allows the head to stay in a bent (flexed) position relative to

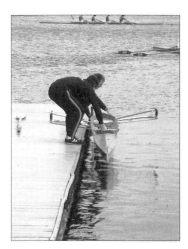
Lifting a boat out of the water is difficult to do correctly

the upper back, effectively letting the neck jut forward. Rowing causes stresses in the spine through the repetitive loaded rotational movement involved, which is the more dangerous if the rower only rows on one side, and has practised intensively through the teenage growth periods. Learning to row on either side and sculling are two ways of reducing the risk of body imbalance due to rowing.

Another risk factor in rowing is lifting the boat in and out of the water. Even the lightest racing shell can seem too heavy when the rower is tired, especially if the boat has taken in water during an outing, and it usually has to be lifted from below the level of the feet, which is a mechanical disadvantage. Rowers are often careless in their lifting technique, not only when handling their boats, but also during weight training, which is an essential background for the sport. Anyone doing weight training as a sport or for fitness training **must** learn correct lifting techniques: failure to do so creates an unacceptably high risk of injury, which is especially likely to affect the spinal joints.

Everyday life and your back and neck

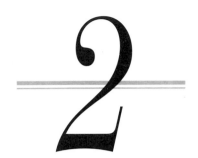

Many back and neck problems arise through sport. However, the pain can then affect normal activities unconnected with sport, interfering with your whole lifestyle. Everyday activities can also be the cause of spinal injuries which then interfere with your sport or fitness exercise. More harm can be done through carelessness in ordinary everyday activities than most people realize. Posture matters: too many problems arise due to poor postural habits, rather than to sports-related or activity-related accidents. Postural problems are largely avoidable. Adults should learn to recognize and correct faults in their posture. Children should be taught from an early age to be aware of their posture and to maintain good posture in every situation. Bad postural habits in children can have damaging long-term effects on the development of the spinal joint structures and their muscles.

There may be times when it is difficult to maintain the theoretically correct posture to protect your spine, due to circumstances beyond your control. If there are problems in your workplace, be prepared to bring them to your employers' notice, with a view to improving the situation and safeguarding your health. Employers should be aware of protecting their workers from injury: working environments should be safe, seating adequate, tasks set according to reasonable patterns, and employees encouraged to look after themselves and keep themselves fit. By and large your posture in any situation is entirely down to you, and you should be conscious of how to look after your spine in the best way possible at all times.

Looking after your back at all hours of the day is absolutely essential for avoiding back problems, recovering from back pain and preventing recurrences. If your practitioner has recommended that you use a corset for your lower back, harness for the upper back, collar for your neck, or any other kind of body support, you should use it strictly according to the instructions. Most body supports, at the very least, remind you to take care to maintain good posture.

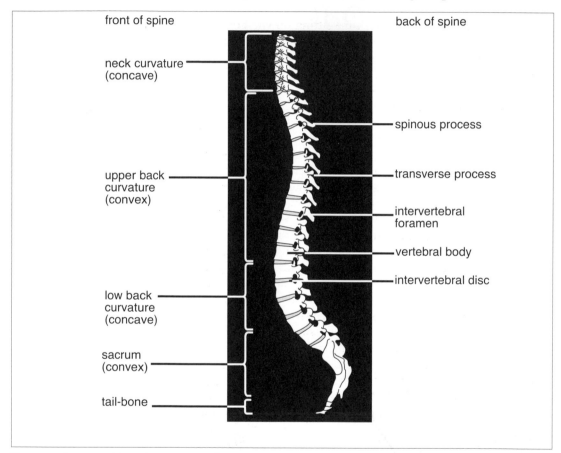

front of spine   back of spine

neck curvature
(concave)

spinous process

transverse process

upper back
curvature
(convex)

intervertebral
foramen

vertebral body

intervertebral disc

low back
curvature
(concave)

sacrum
(convex)

tail-bone

The normal curves of the spine

If you have back or neck pain, everyday chores and pastimes become difficult. You may have to make decisions about whether you should take time off work, which activities you must avoid, how much you can expect to do, and how you can best achieve those tasks which you feel you must do. If you are in doubt, discuss the details of what you want or need to do with your practitioner, and follow any advice given to the letter. You must allocate time every day for the self-help measures and any remedial exercises you have been prescribed: if possible, these should punctuate your day. You may have to re-think your normal programme completely in order to cope with your spinal problem, but you have to remember that the disruption is only temporary, and will be over more quickly if you take care of yourself.

Sitting

Most people spend a lot of their time sitting down. You may not always be able to choose the ideal chair, but you can always decide how you are going to sit. A wheelchair user must have the right size, height and style of chair, with the correct support all round, according to the person's level of disability and functional needs.

Relaxing while sitting down all too often involves letting the back sag and twist into positions which may seem comfortable at the time, but which are very bad for the joints and muscles. Sitting in a slumped position affects your joint structures, especially the little ligaments between the bones, as well as your muscle tone and your circulatory flow. Your spinal ligaments are held fixed in distorted positions. Having adjusted to this, they may feel strained when you try to straighten up again. Your muscle tone drops as you sit still and slumped, so that the longer you sit still, the less your muscles can offer support to the joints. If you remain still, your blood flow slows down, as there is no muscle activity or pressure impulse to stimulate it. For the wheelchair user, frequent shifts of position are essential for stimulating the circulation and preventing pressure sores.

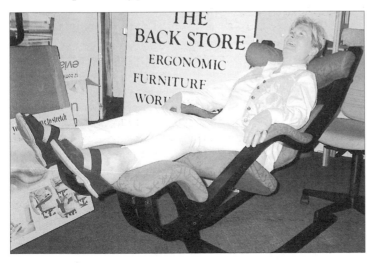

A chair for relaxation: the rocking motion is soothing, and helps to keep joints 'well-oiled'.

A low, soft chair or sofa is especially likely to tempt you into bad posture. The longer you spend in a slumped or twisted position, the worse the overall effect on the back. For instance, watching television for hours on end can leave you with a lot of back stiffness or pain, especially if you have to turn your head to see the screen. It is especially important to stop children from lolling around in adult-sized easy chairs.

If you are suffering from back pain, you must resist the temptation to sit crookedly, even if it feels as though this relieves the pain. Relieving back pain through distorted posture almost always results in an increase of pain when you straighten up again.

Ideally, at rest you should sit on an upholstered upright chair with your back comfortably supported right up to the back of your head. Your lower back should be against the back of the chair, your bottom should be at the same level as your knees or slightly higher, your thighs should be supported, and your feet should be placed on the floor. A low chair makes you slump, forcing your lower back to arch backwards and placing undue strain on the lumbar joints. Tall people often have difficulty finding chairs which are high enough to support them correctly. It is certainly worth investing in a well-designed easy chair if you spend a lot of your leisure time sitting down. Very young children should use chairs of the right height and depth for their size, if at all possible. There are specially constructed chairs which are adjustable so that they 'grow' with the child. Once the child starts school, chairs in the classroom are usually standardized according to age groups. It may be necessary to provide cushion supports or chairs of different sizes to accommodate children of above or below average size.

Any activity or hobby that you do sitting down should be planned so that you can sit in as good a position as possible. The television screen, for instance, should be at eye level or higher straight in front of you, preferably a minimum of several feet away.

Sitting on the floor or sitting up in bed can be bad for the back too. If you sit with your legs straight out, your lower back may be curved backwards, while the muscles, joints and nerves from your pelvis downwards are all stretched and therefore held in tension. If you tuck your legs under you, you twist your hips and lower back into potentially damaging asymmetrical postures. If you want to read in bed, the best position is to move down the bed to lie on your stomach

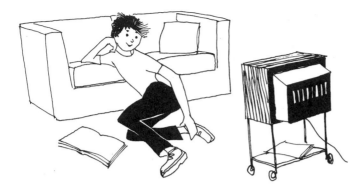

Lolling around for long periods is extremely bad, especially for young backs

with a pillow under your hips, so that the book or paper is in front of you at eye level. Children usually go through phases of wanting to sit in very distorted positions, and they should be gently but firmly discouraged from doing so.

Just as you can decide how you are going to sit, in most circumstances you can also choose how long you spend in one position. Try not to sit still for any length of time. It helps your circulation and the lubrication of your moving joints if you shift your position or get up and walk around at intervals. This is especially important if you watch television, read or do intricate work such as knitting or crocheting, where you might get engrossed for long periods at a stretch if you don't take care to get yourself moving now and then.

Jobs which involve sitting still for long periods, such as supermarket check-out operation, can be especially tiring for both the back and the mind. Most often the chair is a simple swivel seat without full support for the back, shoulder girdles, neck or arms, and the operator has to turn and reach in various directions, as well as handling sometimes heavy items. As all this happens in a very restricted area, it involves a great deal of stress. Frequent 'exercise breaks' should be allowed and encouraged to prevent overuse injuries in such cases.

Bad habits must be curbed. All my patients learn very quickly that they have to obey the cardinal rule of sitting straight and symmetrically when they visit me. I in turn correct my own bad habits, and stop myself from slouching or crossing my legs. I tell my patients off if they sit badly, and they reciprocate by admonishing me if my own posture is less than perfect. The warnings are given lightheartedly, and they serve to remind us all that good posture matters, and that we need to be aware of this at all times.

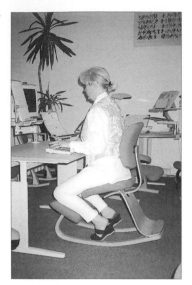

Most modern office chairs are designed for movement to keep the body in good balance and prevent joint stiffness

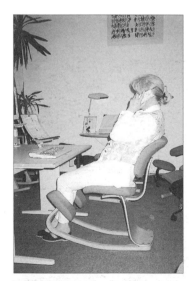

While sitting on the 'kneeling chair' the legs should be relaxed and straightened now and then

Sitting at a desk

Studying, reading and writing should always be done at a table or desk. Sitting on the floor or lying on a bed to read inevitably causes bad, potentially harmful posture.

When you are studying, reading, writing or typing at a desk, you should try to arrange for your body, chair and desk to be in the right relationship to each other. The chair should allow you to sit upright, with your knees slightly lower than your hips, and both feet comfortably on the floor. You may prefer to use a specially formed sloping 'back chair', in which you kneel, or a wedge-shaped cushion to support your hips and knees at the correct angles and to prevent you from crossing your legs. The desk should be high enough to afford room for your legs, and your hands should be slightly lower than your elbows when you are writing or typing. Even if the desk is small, it should be possible to arrange books and papers so that you can refer to them without twisting yourself into awkward shapes.

Sitting still for long periods slows down your general blood flow, and creates cumulative pressures in the joints which bear most of your weight. You should try to adjust your posture frequently while you are sitting. Unless you are using the kneeling type of 'back chair', it helps if your chair has a high back up to neck or head level, so that you can straighten your spine and press your head against the supporting surface. Equally importantly, you should try to get up, walk around and do arm exercises regularly to stimulate the blood flow through your body and tone up your muscles.

On a hard chair, the downward pressure of the weight of your trunk, arms and head is matched by the upward pressure on your seat, because for every force there is an equal and opposite reaction. This creates maximum pressure in the lowest part of your back, complicated by the fact that the hard surface blocks the circulatory flow through your seat to a certain extent. On a softer chair, the pressure is mitigated, and the blood flow is not hindered, so for any job involving sitting for long periods it is best to have a padded but firm chair.

The position of your head is extremely important. Material that you have to refer to while typing is best set up on a stand behind the typewriter, so that you lift your head to look at it, rather than having to look down with your neck bent and twisted. A sloping surface is good for reading and writing by hand. If you have to use papers to one side of you, try to alter the position at intervals during the day, to vary your spinal movements and posture.

If you work at a computer, the screen should be directly in front of you at eye-level, with the keyboard at a comfortable height just below elbow level. Some of the stress on your shoulders and arms can be reduced by having supports to rest your wrists on. Reference or copying material should prefer-ably be on a stand, which you should adjust now and then, to enable you to turn your head in different directions.

If you also have to answer a telephone frequently, you should try to alter its position, so that you do not always turn the same way towards it. Try to alternate hands when you pick up the receiver, to avoid bending your head into the earpiece the same way all the time. If your job involves a lot of telephone work, and you need your hands free for other tasks, you should use headphones rather than a handheld receiver, so that you do not have to tilt your head and neck to hold the receiver.

Standing

Standing still puts pressure on your spine due to the effect of gravity and the weight of your head and trunk. It also causes a reduction in your blood flow, which is due partly to immo-bility and partly to pooling into your legs under the down-ward effect of gravity.

If you have to stand still for long periods in your job, you should try to keep your legs moving at roughly ten-minute intervals. Lifting your heels alternately very slightly off the floor helps your circulation by activating the calf muscles which pump blood through the lower leg, and also by stimu-lating the arch of vessels in your foot. (This is a useful way to stop yourself from fainting if your blood pressure is relatively low and you have to stand to attention, perhaps at a religious ceremony or on parade during military service.) If you are in a position to move your shoulders and arms, especially by lifting your arms upwards, this also helps to relieve the build-up of static pressure on your spinal joints.

As your postural muscles get tired, it becomes harder to stand still and upright, so the shoulders and upper back tend to droop and the pelvis to sag. In jobs like that of shop assis-tant, you should try to walk about or sit down every so often. During each break, try to do some fairly vigorous exer-cises. Alternatively, if you are particularly tired, you should lie down on your back or stomach with your feet raised.

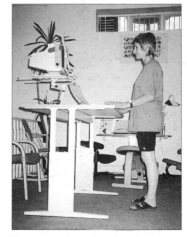

Ergonomically designed desks can be adjusted to allow work standing up

Driving

Whether you are a passenger or the driver, travelling by car can be very uncomfortable and potentially damaging for the spine. Car seats can be beguilingly soft, but if you sink into them with your spine unsupported and have to hold much the same position through a long journey, you can end up with a lot of stiffness and perhaps joint pain. This is worse if you are the driver and the gear-change or the steering wheel is stiff, or at the wrong angle for you to manoeuvre easily. Power steering can help prevent strain through the shoulders, neck and thoracic spine (upper back).

Ideally, your car seat should offer the same kind of support as a good upright chair. Your whole spine should be supported up to the head. Your back should be straight or very slightly reclining. If the back of the seat slants backwards too far, you have to jut your head forwards to see the road ahead. If the front edge of the seat is relatively high and lifts your knees above the level of your hips, your lower back is likely to be held in a backward curve, and your knees and hips are bent, which is a restricting and unfavourable position for them.

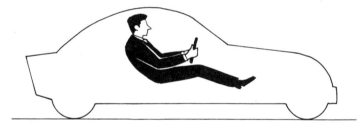

Low-slung sports cars can be hard on the back and neck

When driving, you should be able to rest your head back against the head restraint and still be in control of the steering wheel and gear-change. When you first get into the car, you should sit up as straight as you can in your seat, hold your head high and set the rear-view mirror; if you tend to slump in your seat while driving, you will be reminded to sit up straight again, as the mirror will seem too high. If you have to stretch your arms to reach the steering wheel because your seat is too far away, you create a lot of tension in your neck and shoulders. You should be able to reach the steering wheel without strain, with your shoulders supported against the seat back and your arms slightly bent at the elbows.

It is a great help that so many modern cars have seats which are adjustable in a lot of different directions. One of my most embarrassing moments as a practitioner was having to point out to a patient that he could not drive his very expensive low-slung sports car, as the non-adjustable, virtually horizontal seat held him in entirely the wrong position and was aggravating his back problem. (Fortunately the restriction was temporary as he was cured with treatment and has been able to drive his fast cars with impunity for several years since then.) If your car seat does not allow you to sit correctly, you should be able to improve it in most cases with supports such as lumbar rolls, cushions or specially constructed overlays to provide better support under your seat or behind your back and neck.

If you are a professional driver, whether in a car, taxi, van, truck or lorry, you should work out the best posture for yourself, so that your back is well supported, your shoulders at a comfortable height, and your head reasonably straight. In commercial vehicles, the seat may be fixed and non-adjustable, so you may have to devise supports from cushioning or padding if you cannot find a suitable ready-made back support to fit the seat. Long periods of driving should be avoided, and interspersed with 'exercise breaks', even if you only walk around for a few minutes.

Driving can be tiring and stressful, especially if you do so at night, and this makes it harder for you to motivate yourself to do any kind of exercise when you stop. It can also lead to the situation where you overeat for 'comfort', and so gain weight because your food input exceeds your energy needs. Being overweight of course places extra stress on the spine. One way round this problem is to discipline yourself to start each working shift with a few exercises, which you then try to repeat at each break before you have any refreshments or meals.

If you drive a lot, take care to avoid bad habits in the way you sit. Do you lean sideways to rest your arm on the window ledge? Do you twist your pelvis so that your weight is not evenly balanced over both sides of your bottom? Are your arms over-stretched and tense? Do you let your free leg loll sideways when it is not on the clutch? Try to do a quick mental check of each part of your body now and then, to make sure that you are both comfortable and supported in a good position.

Lifting and manual work

Lifting is a very compressive activity for the spinal joints. Most of us have to lift some loads at some time. We need to

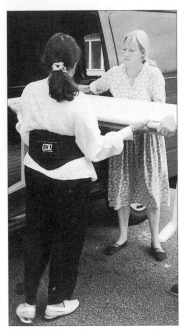

A supportive belt may protect the back while lifting and carrying heavy loads

be fit enough to cope with the load, and we have to be aware of the safest and most efficient lifting technique.

Ideally, to lift any object from the floor, you should bend your knees, grasp the object firmly and keep it close to you as you straighten your legs to bring it up, keeping your back firmly locked straight throughout the movement. This increases the pressure in your abdomen, and helps to protect your spinal joints. Taking a deep breath in before you start the lift, and wearing a support belt both help to increase the intra-abdominal pressure, so it seems they reduce the risk of spinal injury. If you lift even a light object by bending your back and keeping your legs straight, the cumulative pressure on the lower back can amount to more than the discs can tolerate, especially if you have to do repeated lifts. Therefore every object for lifting, however light, should be treated as a weight or load and lifted with due care.

If your job involves heavy lifting, you have to be careful to lift accurately and efficiently at all times. Heavy manual work makes you strong, of course, but at the same time it can contribute to wear and tear degeneration in the spinal joints, especially if you are always doing the same patterns of movement. It is best therefore to try to vary your work, rather than doing one task through the whole working day, to avoid repetitive, cumulative overload on your joints. In building work, if you carry a hod of bricks on your shoulder, make sure you use each shoulder more or less in turn, if you can; if you have to lift large paving stones or flagstones, try to work with a partner; if you handle heavy equipment like a pneumatic drill for breaking up concrete, take frequent breaks; when you have to carry tools or materials, make each load as light and manageable as possible, or get someone to help, or use lifting gear or a forklift truck for very heavy burdens, if possible.

Holiday jobs for youngsters, especially teenagers, can involve lifting very heavy and awkward weights, such as newspapers or milk crates. Employers often think that the teenager is able to cope through being young and strong, but in fact the late teens can be a very vulnerable time for the spine as the hips and spinal bones are going through their final development phases. One of my female patients had taken on a milk round in her early twenties. She managed for about a year before she developed severe back pain, which finally led to her having surgery for a degenerate disc at the age of 33. Two months after the operation, she returned to a

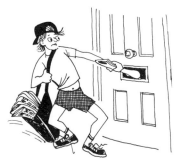

A newspaper round can overload a growing spine

physically demanding job as a waitress. She continued to work out regularly over the next five years in my rehabilitation gymnasium using the Norsk equipment, and had no further problems during this time.

Gardening might be your profession or a hobby, or both. It can place great stresses on the spine, because it often involves quite heavy lifting, as well as repetitive bending and stooping. Except in the case of raised flower beds, window boxes and hanging baskets, most gardening work is done at ground level, below the level of your feet. Planting and weeding require a lot of bending down and twisting movements. Mowing the lawn can be strenuous if the motor mower is heavy and the lawn area large or awkwardly angled. Digging earth is very heavy work, especially if the ground is wet. You should try to use either leg to push the spade into the ground, and alternate your arm positions on the handle so that your trunk does not always twist in one direction as you lift and turn the earth. Seasonal jobs, such as gathering up fallen leaves in the autumn, can be unusually demanding. Even more so are such occasional jobs as chopping wood for logs when a tree has fallen or been cut down.

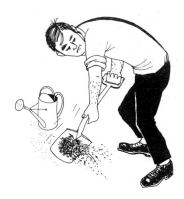

Digging can hurt the back

Never try to do a heavy gardening task all in one go. Give yourself frequent breaks, and spread the job over a few days or weeks if necessary. If you have any doubts about your fitness to take on a particular task, don't do it! Get help or delegate it. Never take risks with jobs which might turn out to be heavier than you anticipated. And never try to finish a job too quickly, especially if you are tired.

Lifting, in everyday life, does not only involve inanimate objects. Animal owners may have to lift their pet if it becomes ill or disabled in some way. Having to lift animals of varying sizes on to a treatment table is an occupational hazard for veterinary surgeons: apart from the weight and awkward shape of the animal, the lifting may be made even more difficult if the animal is struggling. When choosing a pet, it is wise not to take on a large cat or dog which may prove too heavy to handle, if you can choose a smaller animal. When the pet has to be lifted, it should be taken under the back legs and chest, and held close to you, if possible. If the lift is likely to be difficult, it is best to have help. It is important for the animal to keep calm and still, and it helps if your pet has been used to being handled and lifted from an early age. Having to lift the pet is an added reason for not allowing your pet to get overweight through excessive feed-

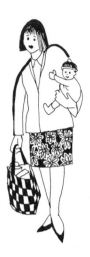

Carrying the baby awkwardly should be avoided

ing and insufficient exercise, besides the other health benefits of keeping your animal as fit as possible.

Lifting people is even more of a problem than lifting animals. The new mother may have suffered back pain during pregnancy or in the course of giving birth. The hormonal changes following the birth quite often make the mother's joints vulnerable to aches and pains, especially in the small hand joints, but also in the sacroiliac joints in the pelvis. The baby normally grows quite quickly during its first few months, so the mother is having to lift, carry and handle an ever-increasing load, perhaps without having recovered fully from the trauma of the birth. The mother may feel constantly fatigued, and therefore in low spirits. If you are in this situation, you must regain good muscle tone quickly, especially in the abdominal muscles, to avoid being at special risk of damaging your back really badly.

In any case, the new mother has to work out the safest ways of lifting and moving the baby around. To avoid problems, you should try to change the way you hold the baby, so that you do not continually stress your spinal joints in the same way. You should also arrange routine tasks such as nappy-changing or bathing the baby so that you do not have to bend over awkwardly. There may be situations when you have to have help. The pram might be too heavy to lift down steps, for instance, or it may be impossible for you to lift and hold a carry-cot.

One of the most practical ways of carrying a small baby is in the harness which you strap in front of you so that the baby's whole body and head are supported over your abdomen and chest. This saves you from walking around with the baby lodged over one of your hips, and has the added advantage of leaving your hands free. As the baby gets bigger, you might use a harness strapped to your back. As the baby gets heavier, you should avoid carrying him or her for any distance. A pushchair should be used for normal transport as soon as the baby can sit up independently.

One of the hardest tasks is to put the baby into a car seat. If the baby seat is on the back seat of a three-door car, you have to lean into it awkwardly, so it is best to avoid this situation if possible. Never try to lift and place the baby quickly, as you need time to position yourself and the baby correctly at each stage of the movement.

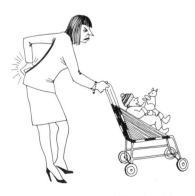

The pushchair should be the right height for the mother as well as the right size for the baby

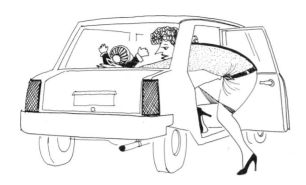

The difficulty of putting the baby into the back of the car

The carer looking after a frail or handicapped adult, or a disabled child, has similar problems to the new mother. You should try to learn the safest and easiest methods of transferring the person from one position to another, or lifting him or her when this is unavoidable. You need to perform these practical tasks in the way that suits you best, but always be aware of protecting your back from harm. Never put yourself at risk by acting too quickly. Prepare yourself and the environment before moving the person in your care.

You must try to arrange the environment so that you and the person you are caring for can move around as easily and safely as possible. Floors should not be slippery or covered in loose small rugs; there should be space to allow for manoeuvring; you should not have to lean over obstacles while trying to support the person; the height of the chair, bed, toilet and bath seat should be at the right level for the person to get on and off without difficulty; safety rails and fixed supports should be installed wherever possible. Most safety elements can be calculated using a little common sense, or learned by experience, but you may also need to seek guidance from your doctor, in the first instance. Qualified practitioners such as physiotherapists, occupational therapists or nurses may also be able to help.

Back problems are an occupational hazard for nurses and physiotherapists when heavy patients need to be lifted and handled. The nurse's task has become much safer since hoists have come into regular use for lifting patients in and out of the bed or the bath. In most countries, strict regulations are coming into force to control the way people like nurses lift patients, for the better protection of all concerned.

Physiotherapists doing manual treatments for heavy and disabled patients have to be conscious of their lifting techniques and spinal posture at all times, to avoid any awkward movement that might cause injury to the therapist, and consequently perhaps to the patient as well.

If heavy lifting is a normal part of your everyday life, there is a strong argument for using a support belt of some kind, to give your lower back some protection. While wearing the belt, it is still important to make sure you lift correctly. Do not let yourself become careless because you think the belt can take the strain. It is important for all manual workers to be properly instructed in safe lifting techniques. There should be monitoring and refresher courses following the initial teaching, to prevent carelessness and short cuts which might be dangerous.

Lifting and carrying bags and cases

Everyday life can involve lifting and carrying heavy loads for work or leisure purposes. Whether for short or long distances, heavy weights in the hands, over the shoulders or on the back can place great compressive stresses on the spinal joints. If the loads are distributed unevenly, the spine is also likely to be twisted and subject to shearing stresses. Back injuries can also be caused if you lift and carry the loads awkwardly, especially if you are not particularly strong or fit, or if you have recently suffered an injury to an arm or leg which makes you compensate with other parts of your body, making you mechanically inefficient.

For the person with a back problem lifting and carrying bags and cases are activities likely to cause further pain and damage. Therefore, it is wise to avoid any kind of lifting and carrying altogether until the back pain is cured.

Because carrying bags can seem like part of normal life, people are often unaware of how ill-prepared they might be for it, and how much harm can be done, if they are relatively unfit. Sometimes the activity is seasonal, as with packing suitcases for holidays, so too little attention is paid to the practical difficulties involved in this 'normal', but not everyday, loading.

For young children, school satchels carried on the back are practical, because they allow for symmetrical distribution of the load and leave both arms free to move. However, once the loads become heavier as the child gets older and has to carry more and bigger books to and from school, any kind of backpack becomes harder to carry safely. The heavier the load, the more the child has to lean forward, bending the lower back and hips to avoid toppling backwards. Young children who do paper rounds, in their early teens or even younger, are often far too small to cope with a big bag of heavy newsprint.

Supermarket shopping must count as one of the most challenging activities for the back. Most people buy trolley-loads of goods in supermarkets, rather than a few items at a time. The trolleys themselves are not yet helpfully designed. As they fill up, they can become difficult to push; and because they are deep, you have to bend down to lift objects out and place them on the conveyor belt at the check-out, only to have to repeat the loading and unloading performance to get the goods out of the store, into your vehicle, and then into your cupboards at home.

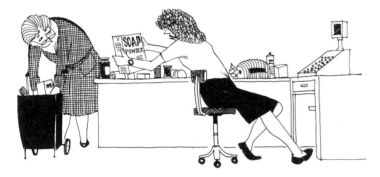

Supermarket shopping can be hazardous for all concerned

One solution to the problem of shopping is to revert to buying smaller amounts at a time. If you carry your shopping in bags, they should be distributed between both arms. However, this places a dragging load on the neck muscles, especially the trapezii which link your neck to your shoulders. Even with relatively small loads, it is better to wheel them home in a shopping trolley.

Bulging brief cases are often very awkward to carry, forcing the bearer to lean to one side while gripping the case with a small handle, or holding it from underneath balanced over one hip. Legal professionals often have to carry huge bundles of documents and books to court.

The professional photographer is usually weighed down with a heavy camera bag which is generally carried over one shoulder, placing sustained compression and shearing stresses on the neck and spine. The situation is worse if the photogra-

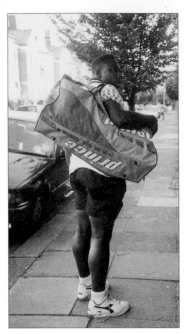

Extra large kit bags can distort the spinal joints

pher has to lug around studio lights, especially up and down stairs or into confined spaces. For television or film cameramen and lighting technicians the situation is even more of a strain, as the cameras and lights are bigger and heavier and often have to be manhandled into difficult positions, for instance on and off trucks or into cramped locations.

Sports bags used to be compact, and indeed some still are. However, many are enormous, designed to hold rackets or bats and several pairs of shoes and changes of clothing. They are bulky, heavy and awkward to carry. If they are slung over the shoulder, they can only be held level if the person leans heavily towards the other side, so that all the joints and muscles of the spine are working at a distinct disadvantage. Golf bags have always been heavy and bulky enough to cause or aggravate back problems. A trolley can help, but it may be difficult to push or pull because the terrain is soft, and on some courses trolleys are not allowed for fear of damaging the turf.

It is particularly unwise to allow a young teenage or preteen player to acquire the habit of carrying a heavily loaded large kit bag which would place undue stresses on immature bones and joints. The problem may not be solved by delegating the bag to a parent, as this may simply be a way of transferring the problem. When a mother told me she had hurt her upper back and shoulder carrying her seventeen-year-old son's cricket bag home for him, I was not impressed by the young man's selfish manners! In any case, it is useful for a youngster to learn to be selective and to carry the minimum kit required, as this lesson can save much wasted effort later on when travelling or moving house.

Suitcase injuries can mar or ruin a holiday. You may have to bend and twist, lifting the load badly, as you place a case into the hold of a coach, on to an overhead rack in a train, or on to the conveyor belt at an airport. This can put your back out, or aggravate an existing back problem. Carrying heavy suitcases is a heavy burden for the shoulders and spine. Apart from compressing the joints, it creates muscle fatigue, especially if you are travelling late at night or when you are tired anyway. For people who have to handle cases all day every day as part of their job, such as airport reception staff, baggage handlers and coach drivers, injury through awkward lifting is a hazard of the job.

It is not always possible to ensure that lifting and carrying bags and cases can be done safely and in the best way possible.

However, there are various factors which can reduce the risk of back problems. These are logical, and only require a basic awareness of your physical capacities, the mechanics of lifting and carrying, and the practical necessities relating to the objects or materials you need to move from one place to another.

Tips for safe lifting and carrying

- Avoid lifting and carrying if your back or neck hurts
- Keep your back straight and use your legs whenever you lift any weight up
- Hold heavy weights close to your body to move them
- Avoid bending over or twisting while holding a weight
- Do not carry heavy weights over long distances
- Carry a heavy bag in each hand or on each shoulder in turn
- If a bag or case is so heavy that you have to tilt your body sideways to balance, divide the load into two smaller bags to hold in each hand
- Young children should not be allowed to struggle with big or heavy loads
- Do not try to lift and carry heavy loads just because you think you *should* be able to manage: be aware of your strength and fitness capacities, and avoid risks
- Share or delegate lifting and carrying if you fear the load might be beyond your strength
- When buying bags or cases, make sure they are suitable for the purpose, and the right size and shape for you to carry, push or pull without undue effort
- Use wheels whenever possible, such as a trolley for boxes or heavy shopping, or a wheeled suitcase for travelling

Housework and cooking

The daily chores of keeping a home clean and tidy can be a nightmare for people with bad backs. I well remember trying to make beds when I had an acute back pain in my late teens, and working out that the only way I could manage was to go round the beds on my knees, tucking in the sheets and blankets as best I could. The fitted sheets and duvets which have come into common use since those days are the best option for easier bed-making.

Moving the furniture around, pushing and pulling the vacuum cleaner, sweeping up, washing or polishing the floor, or reaching to clean into awkward corners, are all activities which involve forcibly twisting and bending the spine. There is an effective resistance if you apply 'elbow grease', or a lot of effort, to clean especially dirty areas or to create a shining polish. You may use heavy electrical equipment, such as a floor polisher. Reaching up above your head places special stress on your neck. Tasks such as fitting or taking down curtains, washing walls, or painting ceilings can cause or aggravate neck problems.

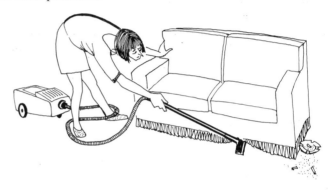

Hazardous housework

Normal housework activities are certainly hard to do without pain if you have a bad back or neck, and they can cause spinal problems, especially if you do a lot of heavy housework when you are tired, or if you do a sudden burst of hard work which you are not used to.The only way to mitigate the strain is to do this kind of work in brief, easy stages, taking very frequent breaks. For jobs which are specially strenuous and take a long time, you should try to use either hand, rather than just your dominant side, if at all possible.

Painting, decorating and do-it-yourself jobs around the home almost invariably take up more time, trouble and effort than you initially bargained for. You have to allow for this in planning any major work, and avoid pressurizing yourself by setting a tight schedule or fixed deadline for completing the work. If you find a particular task difficult, make sure you can call in help to reduce the burden. Never take risks when working around the home. In some situations you have to resign yourself to the inconvenience of living with a half-finished job, rather than risk putting yourself out of action by over-stretching yourself and causing harm.

Serious cooks generally use heavy pots and pans, and may

have to work in a restricted space. You should try to avoid having to lift heavy pans to and from shelves above your head. If you have to bend down to place heavy objects in the oven, dishwasher or cupboard, you must take care to keep your back straight and bend your knees. If it is not possible to move the heavier weights around without jeopardizing or aggravating your back, you should try to get someone to help you. If you regularly cook for a lot of people, it is probably wise to try to use several medium-sized pans, rather than cooking everything together in one giant-sized container.

Work surfaces in the kitchen should be at the correct height, so that you can use them without bending over or having to stretch across them. Storage space should not be over-cluttered, and should be easily accessible. If you spend a lot of time in the kitchen, it is a good idea to reassess your use of the space and change things round as necessary at regular intervals.

Washing and dressing

Washing yourself can become a problem if you have acute or severe back or neck pain. In many situations, you have to bend forwards without being able to use your arms for support. In the normal way, you do the routine daily activities of washing and dressing without paying much attention to how you do them. As they are done almost automatically, you may not even be aware of how you perform most of these tasks, until they become difficult or painful.

It is unusual for these everyday activities to cause pain in themselves, as they do not stress or load the spine unduly. However, it is fairly common for people to experience sudden acute problems while doing them, so that the back or neck suddenly 'goes', for instance, as you bend down to wash your face or put on your socks. There is usually some other reason why this type of spinal problem occurs: the problem may have been building up over time, or there may be some background factor influencing the spinal joints. The slight bending movement might be the 'last straw', proving sufficient to cause a sudden strain in the joints or muscles.

To wash your face and brush your teeth, you usually lean over a basin. To wash your hair, you might bend forwards into the sink, or perhaps backwards if you wash your hair under a shower. These movements generally become painful with any kind of back or neck pain. Reaching down to wash your toes is one of the first tasks to become difficult with even a slight degree of back or neck pain. Washing your back and behind your shoulders is specially hard if you have pain in the upper back. In severe cases of upper back and neck pain, combing or brushing your hair can also become arduous.

When you have a spinal problem, you have to work out the easiest and most efficient ways of keeping yourself clean without aggravating your pain. Sitting down at the sink and using face flannels for washing may be easier than leaning over. You may need to stand up straight to brush your teeth, bending over only for a brief moment when you rinse your mouth out.

In general, it is soothing to have a warm bath, as it stimulates the circulation through your whole body, and relaxes your muscles. Warm baths can help to reduce spinal pain in many cases. Therefore it may be worth trying to have frequent warm baths, even if you normally shower in preference. If you cannot get in and out of the bath easily, you may be able to manage by kneeling to get right down or up. Or a bath seat can help, so that you do not have to sink into or climb out of the full depth of the bath. Alternatively, you may have to settle for showering while you have back or neck pain. If you find you cannot wash your hair without extreme pain, you should try to find a hairdresser with the special facilities for washing hair with the client lying comfortably supported. If you have a severe neck problem with vertebral artery insufficiency (see p.145), it is vital to avoid dropping your head backwards for washing at the hairdresser's, as this may cause sudden loss of consciousness, and can be very dangerous.

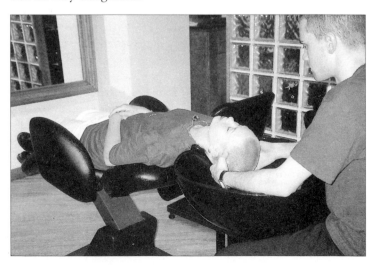

Reclining for the hairwash with the neck supported is ideal for neck pain sufferers

Professionals who deal with the hygiene needs of other people can find themselves working in awkward positions which are not good for the back or neck. Dentists nowadays usually work sitting behind the patient, who is tilted back on a reclining chair. There are similar adjustable chairs and couches for the clients of chiropodists and beauticians. Hairdressers might work standing up or sitting down, and they have to take care to adjust the height of the client's chair so that they can work in the optimum position. Sitting on a mobile stool helps the hairdresser to move around the client easily.

Nurses and carers who attend to the daily needs of a disabled person obviously need to take care when assisting the person into the bath, as this involves potentially heavy loading on the carer's spine. However, it is equally important to be careful while performing the lighter duties of washing and dressing the disabled person, to avoid possibly harmful awkward movements.

Dressing can be problematical for the person with a bad back or neck. Reaching down to put on socks or tights and shoes can become extremely difficult, but you may find you can manage by lying on your back on the bed and bringing each foot towards your hands. If necessary, special gadgets like long-handled shoe horns and stocking aids can be used to reduce the need to reach down to your feet. Pulling a sweater over one's head is hard if the neck or upper back is painful. For ladies with upper back problems, doing up a zip or a bra behind the back can become impossible. To avoid these problems, you might use cardigans or jackets, or front-fastening dresses and bras.

The first priority is to choose clothes which are easy to put on and take off, and comfortable to wear. Tight clothing should be avoided, firstly because it is a struggle to get into and out of, and secondly because it can restrict your circulation and place extra stresses on vulnerable muscles and joints. Remember that if you are attending a practitioner for treatment, you will almost certainly have to remove your outer clothing, down to underwear, for any examination or physical therapy, so be sure to dress in the most practical way possible.

Shoes should also be chosen with care, especially if you walk a lot, or your job keeps you on your feet for long periods each day. Ladies should avoid high heels, as they force the lower back to arch, increasing the lumbar lordosis, and this might cause compression for painful joints. Very flat shoes are not advisable either, as they tend to place a 'drag' on the back of the legs all the way up to the pelvis. The best type of shoe for avoiding or relieving spinal problems, for both males and females, is one with a moderate heel, a firm but flexible sole, and a shock-absorbing insole.

Sex

Sexual activities are a normal part of life for most people who are sexually mature, but they can become problematical if one partner has a bad back or neck. It is important not to allow any practical physical difficulties caused by the bad spine to become major emotional traumas. The back sufferer should not become anxious, and should not be made to feel inadequate. It is also important for the partner to show due sympathy and understanding for the other's pain.

Discussion of any problems is a vital element in solving them. A homosexual patient once confided in me that he felt at least part of his back pain was due to his partner's habit of falling asleep with his knee tucked over the patient's lower back. Every morning, my patient would wake with severe stiffness and pain in his back. This was largely solved by the partners agreeing on a different sleeping position for themselves.

If back pain is severe, the sufferer is unlikely to feel in the mood for sex. This can obviously have negative repercussions in a relationship, if the partner makes an issue of it, or demands sex against the back sufferer's wishes. However, if the desire for sex remains mutual, it is usually possible to work out alternative ways of having sex comfortably and enjoyably.

If a heterosexual couple is trying to conceive, and the woman is suffering from back pain, it is probably wise to delay starting the pregnancy until her back has recovered. As back pain in females sometimes relates to hormonal change, it is possible that a particular episode of back pain might be linked to coming off the contraceptive pill. Time is needed to allow for adjustment. In all cases, it is vital for the female to be as fit and strong as possible before the pregnancy, to avoid problems during and after childbirth. Protective back exercises, preferably under the guidance of an obstetric physiotherapist, should be maintained throughout the whole period of pregnancy and afterwards, if at all possible.

Sleeping

Patients often ask if there is a special bed they should buy to help a bad back or to prevent back problems. This is an extremely difficult question to answer, as there is no single style of bed which suits every type of back problem, or which can be guaranteed to prevent trouble. It is not always necessary to change your bed just because you have suffered a back problem, but it is essential to think of doing so if your symptoms are worst during the night or first thing in the morning. If you find that a change of beds helps your back problem, then you should try to work out what kind of bed is better for you than your own.

Should you have a bed custom-made for you? This is difficult to say, as there are no hard and fast criteria which specify that a mattress and base constructed in a certain way must necessarily help. On the other hand, they might. Then again, it is possible that as your back problem recovers you can sleep comfortably in your old bed again, so the need to change beds may only be temporary.

Most often, the search for a suitable bed has to be resolved according to what you find suits you. There is little doubt that a very soft bed which has sagged in the middle is likely to create or aggravate back problems, because it not only offers no support at all to the middle of your body, which is the heaviest part, but also drags your lower back into a bent and twisted position. On the other hand, a very hard bed can create back stiffness and pain through not allowing the spinal joints to relax into their normal contours during sleep.

The best general solution is to have a moderately firm mattress on a slatted wooden base. But some individuals with back pain do better with a soft mattress, others with a very firm mattress, others with a futon on the floor. The final decision may depend on trial and error. It is always important to remember to turn your mattress at regular intervals, according to the supplier's instructions, unless the bed is specifically designed so that this is not necessary.

Another question is whether there is a special way to lie in order to be in the correct position overnight. My own feeling is that sleep is a natural activity, and you should sleep in whatever position you find comfortable. Sleeping positions vary according to individual preference, some people lying prone (on their stomachs), others on one side or the other, some on their backs. Generally speaking, it is better for your neck if you use one soft pillow, but some people prefer two thin pillows, others no pillow at all. During sleep, you turn over and move automatically, and it is important not to impede your natural pattern, as this can create tension. However, you may find it helpful to try one of the relaxation positions using one pillow for your head and extra pillows to support your limbs.

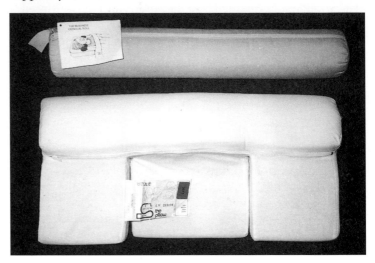

A special pillow or neck roll can help to relieve neck pain

Tips for minimizing or avoiding back pain in everyday life

- Avoid any activities which you know might cause pain
- Avoid over-tiring yourself
- Allow time for rest and relaxation every day
- Do your remedial exercises frequently and regularly
- Always try to sit and stand correctly
- Avoid being still in any position for long periods
- Do not do physically demanding or repetitive tasks over long periods of time
- Get help with tasks that might be too difficult for you or delegate them
- Prioritize your activities: leave out those which are risky
- Plan ahead, to avoid problems
- Report any problems to your practitioner
- Never go against the advice of your practitioner

Structure and functions of the back and neck

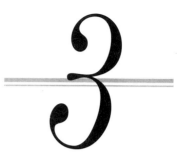

The spine consists of bones called vertebrae, joint capsules, ligaments, discs, blood vessels, tendons, muscles, nerves and the spinal cord. It extends from the neck (cervical spine) down to the tailbone (coccyx). It is very closely linked to the pelvis in its structure and function, not to mention in injury. Therefore any description of the spine usually includes the back of the pelvis as well.

It is extremely unlikely that anyone can boast of having a 'perfect' spine. It would also be difficult, if not impossible, to define what a perfect spine should be like, or how it should look, feel and function. Because the structure of the spine is so complicated, there are innumerable variations on the basic structure in individuals. Differences from the theoretical norm include extra or deficient vertebrae, variations in the shapes of the bones, and tight or lax ligaments or muscles.

THE BONES OF THE BACK, NECK AND PELVIS

The spinal column is divided into sections. There are normally seven vertebrae in the neck (cervical spine), twelve in the upper back (thoracic or dorsal spine) and five in the low back (lumbar spine). The lumbar spine rests on the pelvic basin, a structure consisting of the sacrum, tailbone (coccyx), two flank-bones (ilia or innominate bones) and the pubic bones. All the bones comprising the vertebral column are numbered from above downwards, so that the top neck vertebra is called C1 (first cervical vertebra) while the lowest bone in the low back is L5 (fifth lumbar vertebra). Although the sacrum is a single bone in which the separate parts are fused together, it is still described as S1 to S5, as the previously distinct vertebrae can still be identified in the shape of the bone.

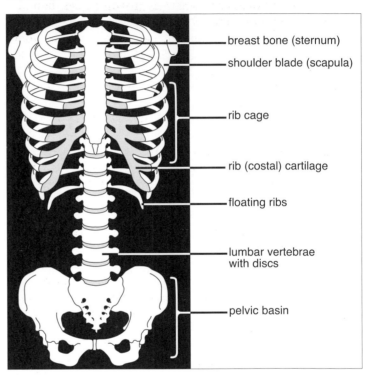

breast bone (sternum)

shoulder blade (scapula)

rib cage

rib (costal) cartilage

floating ribs

lumbar vertebrae with discs

pelvic basin

The bones of the spine, rib cage and pelvis

Bone growth and development

All the bones of the body grow by stages. Before birth, the various cells from which the different bones start their development process begin to multiply inside the embryo. Each part of every bone develops from a special growth point, technically called a centre of ossification. Most bones start out in a soft form and are mainly cartilage at first, gradually transforming into hardened bone during the first few years of life. The final shape and size of each bone are acquired from secondary centres of ossification which develop at different periods for different bones. An epiphysis is the end part of a bone which forms the joint surface with a neighbouring bone. It is separated from the main part of its bone by an epiphyseal plate (growth plate or growth cartilage), which allows for active bone growth until maturity is reached. Where tendons or muscles join on to bones the growth points are usually called apophyses.

The process through which different parts of a bone come together to produce the mature, finished shape is called fusion. The bones grow throughout childhood and the teen years, but some bones complete their growth earlier than others. In the vertebrae, the secondary centres for ossification appear at around puberty, and the parts finally fuse by about the age of 25, the same period in which the flank-bones (ilia) become fully formed. In the sacrum, ossification is generally complete by the age of 20, although the central parts of the bone may remain unossified until later in middle age. The coccyx ossifies relatively late, and may not become a fully united bone until the age of 30. While a bone is going through its fusion phase, it is especially vulnerable to overuse injury, whether from repetitive jarring stresses or shearing due to the pull of the muscle or tendon attached to the bone.

The vertebrae

In most of the vertebrae, the main elements forming each bone are the vertebral body, laminae, spinous process, transverse processes, pedicles, and superior and inferior articular processes. However, the vertebrae are not identical to each other. Each reflects the special function it performs according to its position in the vertebral column. The cervical vertebrae, for instance, are much finer than the lumbar vertebrae which are the biggest and strongest of the column because they have to support much more load. The thoracic vertebrae are characterized by special indentations for the ribs on the sides of their bodies and their transverse processes.

In the majority of vertebrae, the vertebral body is the main block of bone, cylindrical in shape, which gives the backbone most of its height and forms its solid basic structure. Behind each body is the vertebral arch, which is composed of struts of bone joined up to form a kind of ring behind the vertebral body. The space it creates is known as the vertebral canal, within which lies the spinal cord. The pedicles are small projections of bone from the back of the vertebral body. They are paired, one on each side of the midline of the vertebral body. The laminae are continuations of the pedicles, and project backwards in pairs to meet and form the spinous process. Where the pedicles and laminae meet, they support the transverse processes, which jut out sideways from the ring of the vertebral canal, and the superior and inferior articular processes (zygapophyses), which project upwards and downwards respectively.

The transverse processes in most of the neck (cervical) vertebrae lie beside the vertebral bodies rather than behind, and they form an arch on either side to protect the vertebral arteries and veins. Most of the cervical spinous processes form double end-points (technically they are called bifid) rather than one as in the thoracic and lumbar vertebrae. The top two cervical vertebrae are totally different from all the others. The first cervical vertebra, the atlas, which supports the head (cranium), is simply a ring of bone without a body. The axis underneath it has a small body but is uniquely characterized by its odontoid process, a stub of bone which projects upwards to provide a secure joint with the atlas.

Apart from the normal functional differences between the vertebrae at different levels in the spine, there may be individual variations in spinal structure. Some people have an extra lumbar vertebra, technically called a transitional vertebra, making six instead of five. Others might have a degree of fusion between the sacrum and the fifth lumbar vertebra, technically known as sacralization, which reduces the functioning lumbar vertebrae to four. Sometimes parts of the bones are imperfectly formed, showing visible defects on X-ray. With age, the effects of wear and tear or injury can create slight deformities at the edges of the vertebral bones. Osteophytes are protrusions from bones which are usually caused by irritation of the bone surface, and which generally appear at the edges of joints. In the facet (zygapophyseal) joints, the inner, front parts of the joint surfaces may become thicker with age, while there may be thinning and splitting of the cartilage on the bone surfaces in the back parts. There is often a loss of bone density with age, especially in females going through the menopause. This gradually makes the spine shorter by causing a narrowing of the vertebral bodies, so that in very old age a person may become significantly shorter than before.

The vertebral bodies are deep-seated, so you cannot feel them by pressing your back with your hands. However, you can feel the spinous processes of the vertebral column almost all the way up from the sacrum to the neck. The most prominent spinous processes are at the base of the neck and the top of the upper back, technically C7 and T1. It is much harder to feel the facet joints and transverse processes to the sides of the vertebral column, as they are well covered by the spinal muscles, especially when you are standing up, but you can just make them out if you press in deeply enough, the more easily if you are lying on your stomach.

The pelvis and hips

The lowest lumbar vertebra rests on top of the sacrum, a wedge-shaped bone which forms the central part of the pelvic basin. Below the sacrum, the tailbone (coccyx) consists of four tiny vertebrae more or less fused together. On either side of the sacrum lie the flank- or hip-bones (technically the ilia or innominate bones), which are bound to the sacrum at the sacroiliac joints, and whose front parts form the pubic bones, which are bonded together at the symphysis pubis. At each side of the flank-bone is a specially formed cup (technically acetabulum) which forms the socket for the head of the thigh-bone at the hip joint. Because the hip joints and the sacroiliac joints are structurally interdependent, movements of the hips have an effect on the low back. Leg-length differences can affect the balance between the hips and the way they move. This is why differences in the lengths of your legs can be significant in back problems.

The pelvic basin and hip flexor muscles

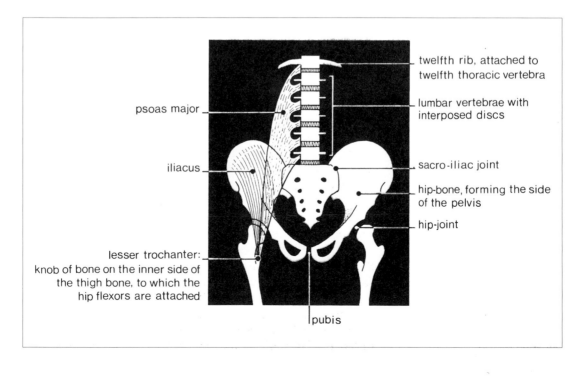

psoas major

iliacus

lesser trochanter:
knob of bone on the inner side of
the thigh bone, to which the
hip flexors are attached

twelfth rib, attached to
twelfth thoracic vertebra

lumbar vertebrae with
interposed discs

sacro-iliac joint

hip-bone, forming the side
of the pelvis

hip-joint

pubis

You can feel the iliac crests along the tops of the hip-bones if you run your fingers along them on either side of your body just below your waist. If you press your fingers under the centre of one buttock while you are sitting down, you can feel the seat-bone (ischial tuberosity). It is harder to feel the seat-bone while you are standing up, because it is well covered by the thick buttock muscles (mainly gluteus maximus and the attachment point of the hamstrings). The sacrum is the hard, flattened surface you can feel centrally in the lowest part of your back. At the tip of the sacrum you can feel the tailbone, which lies between the buttocks. The sacroiliac joints form irregular lines on either side of it, slanting inwards towards the tailbone. You can feel and see the upper ends of the sacroiliac joints as prominent dimples just above the main contours of the buttocks. The pubic bones and symphysis are easily palpable if you press your fingers into the centre of your groin and slightly to either side.

THE JOINTS OF THE SPINE

From the second cervical vertebra downwards, each vertebra is linked to the next through several separate joints. The vertebral bodies are linked to each other through the intervening intervertebral discs, and these are classified as cartilaginous joints, which means that they do not contain any fluid-producing lining. The laminae are connected to each other in fibrous joints, again without a synovial lining, and the transverse and spinous processes are similarly interconnected. All these joints are known technically as syndesmoses. The articular processes interlink to form synovial joints, which means that they are covered by an enclosing capsule with a fluid-producing (synovial) lining to provide lubrication for smooth movements. The joints formed by the articular processes are called zygapophyseal or facet joints.

Between each pair of vertebral bones is a gap, technically known as an intervertebral foramen. Such gaps lie on either side behind the vertebral bodies between the joints formed by the posterior arches, and they form a kind of tunnel allowing the spinal nerves to pass out of the spinal column.

In the upper back (thoracic spine) the ribs are attached to each side of the thoracic vertebrae. The tip of each rib is connected to the side of a disc between two vertebral bodies, and to special grooves in the bones just above and below the disc, forming a synovial (fluid-filled) joint. Except for the eleventh and twelfth ('floating') ribs, each rib is also attached in a synovial joint to the transverse process which juts out sideways from the vertebral body.

The sacrum is attached to the flank-bone (ilium) on either side to form the two sacroiliac joints, which are synovial, as they have a fluid-forming lining within the capsule which encloses the joint. The pubic symphysis is formed where the pubic bones meet at the front of the pelvic basin. This is a fibrocartilaginous joint formed by a disc between the two bones, which are also linked by strong ligaments.

Ligaments

All the joints in all the regions of the spine are bound by ligaments which limit their movement in certain directions. Many ligaments are specially thickened parts of the joint capsules which surround synovial joints. Others form direct connections between two bones. Ligaments are soft bindings, technically made of collagen, and organized in bundles as dense regular connective tissue. They cannot contract as a tendon can. They are only slightly elastic, but they are capable of yielding and regaining their shape under a normal amount of tension. If they are being stretched beyond the normal limit, they are protected by surrounding muscles which react reflexly by contracting to help prevent further stretching. However, if the protective mechanisms fail to prevent serious over-stretching, the ligaments strain or tear.

The whole vertebral column is bonded by two long ligaments, the anterior longitudinal ligament which is attached to the front of the vertebral bodies and discs from the base of the skull to the front of the top of the sacrum, and the posterior longitudinal ligament which is indirectly linked to the base of the skull and passes down behind the vertebral bodies and discs from the second cervical vertebra to the sacrum. The anterior longitudinal ligament protects the vertebrae from excessive backward movement when you bend backwards, and the posterior longitudinal ligament prevents excessive separation of the vertebral bodies when you bend forwards.

The facet (zygapophyseal) joints are held together by the joint capsules which surround each joint. All the syndesmoses behind the vertebral bodies have strong ligaments binding the bones to each other. The ligaments are named according to their position: the interspinous ligaments bind each vertebral spine to the next, the ligamentum nuchae links the outer tips of the spinous processes in the neck, the supraspinous ligament binds the tips of the spinous processes from the seventh cervical vertebra downwards, and the intertransverse ligaments lie between the transverse processes. The laminae which project backwards to form the spinous processes are connected to each other by relatively elastic ligaments called the ligamenta flava (yellow ligaments).

The ribs are held in place at the costovertebral joints by the joint capsules, reinforced by ligaments. Except for the 'floating' ribs, the outer attachment of each rib at its costo-transverse joint is also bonded by a separate ligament to the transverse process above itself.

The sacroiliac joint is held together by the extremely strong sacroiliac ligament, which consists of three parts, the front, middle and back, technically called the ventral, interosseous and dorsal sacroiliac ligaments. The central portion is the strongest. Apart from the long ligaments which connect the sacrum to the vertebral column, the lowest lumbar bone, L5, is bound to the flank-bone (ilium) on either side by the iliolumbar ligament. This is another extremely strong ligament, but only in the adult, as it does not become properly formed until after childhood.

The intervertebral discs

Cushioning discs lie between each pair of vertebrae from the top of the sacrum at the back of the pelvis up to the second cervical vertebra. There is no disc between the atlas and axis (first and second vertebrae in the neck), or between the atlas and the base of the skull. The twenty-three discs make up about one fifth of the total length of your backbone (vertebral column). They are thickest in the low back (lumbar spine) and thinnest towards the top of your upper back (thoracic spine). In the low back and neck (cervical spine) the discs are thicker in their front parts than at the back, in keeping with the curves in these areas. In the upper back the discs are roughly the same thickness from front to back.

In all areas of the spine the discs are tied to the ligaments in front of and behind the vertebral bodies, and attached to the hyaline cartilage which covers the flat upper and lower bone surfaces of the vertebral bodies. (This type of cartilage is a special form of bone covering, not quite as hard as bone itself, but not to be confused with the kind of soft buffering cartilages or menisci which you find in the knees, for instance.) In the upper back, the discs are also linked by ligaments to the heads of the ribs.

Each disc has a soft fluid central part, the nucleus pulposus, with a firmer outer part around it, the annulus fibrosus. The nucleus pulposus does not lie in the centre of the disc, but closer to the back of the structure, and it is especially well developed in the low back and neck, less so in the upper back. From birth, the nucleus pulposus is very large, soft and jelly-like, but it gradually becomes harder and less fluid from about the late teen period onwards, so that its water-binding properties and elasticity are progressively reduced. The annulus fibrosus is laminated, formed in bands which are interwoven in a complicated pattern. It has an inner part of fibrocartilage and a thinner outer section of collagenous tissue. It retains the nucleus pulposus securely within its structure, and provides stability through its connections with the surrounding bones. It is also elastic enough to help the shock-absorbing actions which are mainly performed by the nucleus pulposus.

Each disc has a covering over its upper and lower surfaces called the vertebral end-plate, which separates the disc from the vertebrae above and below it, and consists of hyaline cartilage and fibrocartilage. At birth and through early childhood, the end-plate forms part of the growth plate of the nearest vertebral body, but as the growth processes slow down in the late teens the end-plate becomes less closely attached to the vertebral body, while remaining strongly bonded to the disc. From the age of about 20 onwards, the end-plate gradually becomes thinner and weaker, and its outer cartilage cells tend to die off in older age.

The blood supply to each disc is limited, as only the very outer parts of the annulus fibrosus receive nutrition from blood vessels. Otherwise the discs do not have their own blood supply (technically they are *avascular*) and they depend on diffusion of nutrient fluids from their neighbouring bones. Most of the fluid and nutrition exchange is done through the nucleus pulposus. As the vertebral end-plate is gradually sealed off from the vertebral body, it loses its ability to allow the passage of nutrients through to the nucleus pulposus, and this can contribute to the progressive age-related degeneration of the nucleus.

THE SPINAL CORD AND PERIPHERAL NERVES

The brain controls virtually every aspect of our activities, awareness and feelings. Some activities take place at a conscious level, such as hitting a tennis ball, whereas others, such as the beating of the heart, happen automatically. The part of the nervous system through which we control our voluntary movements is called the somatic system, and the automatic part is called the autonomic nervous system. Both systems work by transmitting information and messages in each direction between the outlying parts of the body and the central nervous system which consists of the brain and spinal cord.

The nerves which are formed from the spinal cord and which supply every area of the body outside the central nervous system are known as the peripheral nervous system. The peripheral nervous system supplies sensation nerves to all parts of the body, as well as motor nerves which control muscle actions.

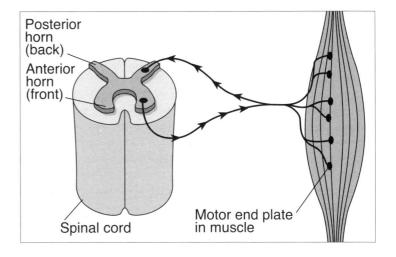

Posterior horn (back)

Anterior horn (front)

Spinal cord

Motor end plate in muscle

A motor nerve linking the spinal cord to a muscle. Simplified, messages to the muscle are sent from the anterior horn, while messages from the muscle go into the posterior horn of the spinal cord

The main difference between the central and peripheral nervous systems is that peripheral nerves are capable of regenerating even after they have been totally severed, whereas the cells of the central nervous system cannot recover once they have been destroyed by illness or injury. A bad accident which completely shatters the spinal cord leaves the victim paralysed in the area below the level of the break. A stroke or head injury which causes some brain damage may cause problems in controlling the movements in one side of the body. (However, even in the case of quite bad brain damage, modern research has shown that, although the brain cells cannot mend themselves, they are capable of adapting, so it is still possible to regain some function.)

The nervous system is a very complicated series of mechanisms. All the interrelated parts, and especially the nutrition elements and blood supply, have to be functioning properly for the nervous system to work accurately. Any interference or damage to the peripheral nervous system can cause a variety of symptoms from pain, strange skin sensations such as tingling or numbness, abnormal feelings of heat or cold, loss of muscle power, and loss of co-ordination.

The spinal cord (technically known as the neuraxis or the medulla spinalis) is part of the central nervous system, and at its upper end it leads into the lowest part of the hindbrain, the medulla oblongata. It stretches downwards within the spinal canal, ending at about the level of L2, or sometimes slightly higher up. Below the level of L2 a thin filament formed of connective tissue and called the filum terminale continues downwards from the end of the spinal cord to the top of the tailbone (coccyx). The spinal cord is protected by three layers of membranes (technically meninges). Cerebrospinal fluid, which is essential for both the nutrition of the spinal cord and its ability to glide smoothly during movements of the backbone, is contained between the middle membrane, the arachnoid mater, and the inner one, the pia mater. The dura mater is the tough outer protective layer, and it has specially thickened extensions which act as sleeves covering the roots of the spinal nerves where they leave the spinal cord.

There are 31 pairs of spinal nerves, 8 in the neck (cervical nerves), 12 in the upper back (thoracic), 5 each in the low back (lumbar) and sacrum (sacral), and 1 in the tailbone (coccygeal). They are attached to each side of the spinal cord, and pass out between the bones of the spine through special channels called intervertebral foramina. They lie behind the intervertebral discs and adjoining vertebral bodies, in front of the facet (zygapophyseal) joints, and between the bone pedicles which lie above and below the nerves as they emerge at any given level of the spine. As the spinal cord is shorter than the backbone, the lowest spinal nerves spread downwards from the end of the cord to their separate exit points in a bunch of nerve strands called the cauda equina (horse's tail).

Each spinal nerve is formed from two distinct parts, the anterior and posterior roots (ventral and dorsal rami), which come away from the front and the back of the spinal cord respectively. The cervical nerves supply the skin and muscles of the neck itself, the chest, upper back, arms and hands. The upper two (anterior) thoracic nerves also supply the arms, but mainly they supply the middle part of the upper back, the rib cage and the abdominal wall. The lumbar nerves supply the lowest part of the abdominal wall and trunk, the groin and hip regions, the legs and the feet. The sacral nerves supply the lowest parts of the back.

The main nerves in the arms and legs are formed from several spinal nerves which join together, although each splits into fine divisions, rather like telephone wires, to reach every part of the area being supplied. The biggest peripheral nerve in the body is the sciatic nerve, which consists of the anterior parts of the nerves from L4 to S3. From the low back it travels downwards to supply the back of the thigh and the knee, splitting into two parts below the knee to provide for the lower leg, ankle and foot. The femoral nerve supplies the front of the thigh, and arises from the anterior parts of L2 to L4. In the arm, the median nerve is formed from C5,6,7,8 and T1 to supply the central region of the front of the arm and hand. The ulnar nerve, from C8 and T1, passes down the inner side of the arm, forearm and hand, and winds behind the inner side of the elbow, called the 'funny bone' because of the strange sensation you feel if you hit the bone and its accompanying nerve. The radial nerve is the biggest in the arm, arising from C5, 6, 7 and 8, and it supplies the back of the upper arm, forearm and hand.

Although it is possible to identify the nerve roots which form the main nerves, there is a lot of overlap, so that various nerves can influence the same regions. Individuals also vary in the way their nerve pathways are constructed. This is why it is not always easy to identify which nerve root or spinal segment might be involved in particular pain patterns arising from back or neck problems.

BASIC FUNCTIONS OF THE BACK AND NECK

The overall structure of the back and neck allows for three major uses: protection, support, and leverage for movement.

Protection

One of the primary functions of the spine and pelvis is to provide a kind of 'armour' of bones to protect delicate structures from damage.

The spinal bones surround the spinal cord which, together with the brain forms the central nervous system. The spinal cord is encircled within the arches of bone formed at the back of the central blocks (bodies) of the vertebral column. It is securely held, and it takes a very severe injury to break the protective bone circles sufficiently to cause damage to the spinal cord.

Equally importantly, special rings of bone at the sides of the vertebral bones in the neck enclose the arteries and veins to protect the vital passageway for blood between the heart and the brain. If these blood vessels are blocked in any way, whether through injury to the neck or disease in the blood vessels themselves, you will feel dizzy or light-headed. In some types of neck problem, you may find that tilting your head a certain way causes these symptoms.

Important parts of the digestive system and the female reproductive organs are secured within the pelvic basin which surrounds them from the back and sides. The abdominal muscles provide a firm and active control mechanism in front of the body. The heart and lungs are encased behind the breast-bone (sternum) and inside the rib cage, which is linked to the bony arches of the spinal column.

Support

The vertebral column and the pelvic basin are essential supporting structures for the body. Without its bony framework, the human body would be jelly-like. A new-born baby has only the soft beginnings of a bone structure, and so seems very pliable. Before the neck has developed, there is no stable bony or muscular support for the head, so anyone handling a baby during the first weeks of life has to take care to support the head and prevent it from falling backwards, as this might damage the nerve, blood and breathing systems which travel down the neck.

As soon as the bones develop, together with their binding joint structures, muscles and tendons, the body acquires its basic framework for stability. It is then able to provide a base of support for active movements, allowing some muscles to contract in order to move one or more joints, while others relax so as not to oppose the movement, and still others

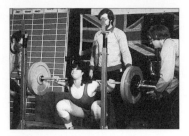

The Valsalva manoeuvre: before lifting a heavy load, the powerlifter takes a deep breath and holds it during the effort of lifting

remain in tension to keep parts of the body which are not involved in the movement still or relatively still.

Ever since human beings became upright rather than four-legged, the spine has had to act as the stable connection holding up the trunk, shoulder girdle and head against the effect of gravity. The weight of your skull and brain is supported on your neck bones whenever you are upright. In standing, the load of your head, upper body and trunk is transmitted along the spine, through the hips and legs, and down to the feet. When you sit down, the whole load of your head and upper body is borne by the lowest part of your spine and pelvis, because the chair acts as an equal and opposite force upwards against the weight. A soft chair or cushion dissipates this upward counter-pressure up to a point, whereas a hard chair maximizes it.

The intervertebral discs are designed to act as shock absorbers, providing relatively soft and adaptable cushioning between the rigid bones of the spine. Apart from their mechanical functions, the intervertebral discs provide a source of fluid and nutrition exchange between each disc and the vertebrae on either side of it.

When the spine is subjected to mechanical stresses, the discs effectively distribute the stresses outwards, so that they can be absorbed. The healthy disc is quite elastic and resilient, so it can recover immediately from forces which compress it. Pressures inside the discs vary according to several factors. The pressures in your lower discs rise if you are sitting down, especially if your back is hunched. The pressures also rise when you bend over forwards or sideways, and especially during heavy lifting, the more so if you hold your breath in the Valsalva manoeuvre (see p.214). Disc pressures are lower when you are standing up, when you keep the curve of your low back arched in extension (maintaining the lumbar curve), and when you twist your spine to either side. The pressures are lowest when you lie down on your back or stomach.

In children and young people under the age of sixteen, the intervertebral discs are stronger than the bones on either side of them, and the rise in pressure in the discs when they are under load is less than in adult discs. Therefore the bones are more likely to be damaged in an accident to a young person, and it takes an extremely violent force, usually involving forward bending, to damage the discs themselves.

Although the healthy disc is capable of absorbing a great

deal of pressure, discs which have degenerated as a result of injury, 'wear and tear' or ageing processes show altered pressure changes under loading, and are less capable of dissipating stresses.

Leverage for movement

The spine allows the trunk to bend forwards and backwards, to lean sideways, and to twist to either side. The freedom of movement in each direction is dictated or limited by the shape of the bones which interact, the formation of the joint capsules, the size, strength and direction of the surrounding ligaments and muscles, and the intervertebral discs. The movements possible in each individual joint of the vertebral column are very small, but overall an adequate range of movement for our functional needs is provided by the combination of movements available in the co-ordinated joints of the spine.

The neck has special flexibility, letting the head tilt, twist and bend in various directions from the starting point of facing forwards. The thoracic spine, or upper back, is specially constructed to allow for a good range of twisting (rotatory) movements, whereas it is restricted in bending forwards, backwards and sideways. The rib joints which are attached to the edges of the thoracic vertebrae have a small degree of twisting and gliding movement, which allows your rib cage to expand when you take a deep breath. The shoulder blades slide around the back of the chest, and co-ordinate movements between the shoulders, thoracic spine and rib cage.

The low back (lumbar spine) has greatest freedom in moving forwards (into flexion), less for leaning backwards (into extension) and least for twisting (rotation). Forward bending is limited by the way the bones of the facet (zygapophyseal) joints come together, the amount of stretch or tightness in the ligaments and muscles along the spine, and the intervertebral discs. Backward bending and twisting are both limited, especially by the bone shapes and the way in which the protruding parts of the bones come together.

The pelvis forms the lowest supporting structure to the trunk. The pubic joint in front and the two sacroiliac joints behind are very tightly bound, although the sacroiliac joints are capable of slight shearing movements. The pelvis as a whole basically functions as a unit, tipping forwards and backwards or tilting sideways.

The trunk has some involvement in virtually all movements of the arms and legs. It provides a base for movements of the limbs: these can be co-ordinated more or less symmetrically between the limbs, as in running, swimming and sculling, or in varied patterns of movement, as in racket games, field hockey and fencing.

On either side of the pelvis are the connections with the thigh bones which form the hip joints. Movements at the hips are closely connected to movements in the lowest part of the trunk, and automatically involve some activity in the pelvis when we are standing up. In a much looser connection, the upper spine links to the arms by way of the shoulder girdle, which consists of the collar bone (clavicle), shoulder blade (scapula) and arm bone (humerus). Because the shoulder joint is the most mobile in the body, we can move our arms without necessarily involving the spine directly. However, when we use our arms, even if the trunk is not involved in the movement itself, some of the trunk muscles normally come into play to stabilize the neck, chest and spine.

All the active movements of the back and neck which you can perform at will are achieved by muscles which pull the bones into the various directions which you choose.

MUSCLES IN THE BACK AND NECK

Traditionally, muscles were described as having a starting-point, or origin, and ending-point, or insertion. Muscles were considered to act primarily from the origin, pulling the insertion towards it. Nowadays, the technical descriptions have been modified, as it is recognized that the way nerves activate muscles is more complicated than was previously thought, and that most muscles can work from either end, so that they do not necessarily perform actions which can be strictly classified as primary or secondary.

There are many muscles extending along the back from the pelvis to the skull which control the movements of the head, neck and trunk backwards, sideways and into rotation. Many of the vertebral joints, especially in the neck, also have small localized muscles which perform specific movements. Technically, back muscles are defined according to their nerve supply, so that muscles which receive their nerve supply from the posterior parts (dorsal rami) of the spinal nerves are true back muscles, while those which take their nerves from the anterior parts (ventral rami) are considered to be intermediate, and functionally comparable to the muscles which control rib movements.

Muscle functions

Muscles which create joint movements are technically voluntary muscles, as opposed to the involuntary muscles which work automatically, like the heart. The voluntary muscles are attached to the bones on either side of the moving part of the joint. Muscle work which results in joint movement is called *isotonic* or *dynamic*. The simplest type of joint movement occurs when one end of a muscle shortens to pull the bone in a certain direction against gravity or a resistance, while the other end fixes the bone on the other side of the joint. Technically this is called a *concentric* contraction. In fact, muscles do not work singly in isolation, but in groups. While one muscle group works, there are usually other groups working as well, some paying out (technically *synergically*) to allow the movement to happen, and some acting as fixators or stabilizers, to prevent unwanted movements in related joints. Muscle contraction which does not create noticeable joint movement is called *static* or *isometric* work. You can perform isometric muscle contractions by pressing your hands together or pushing your head backwards against a fixed headrest.

All active muscle work done against gravity or a resistance involves a shortening in the working muscles as they contract to create joint movement. The reverse movement requires the muscles to lengthen out. If you do the reverse movement slowly, with control, you work the muscles *eccentrically*. This is an extremely important type of muscle work following injury. It is harder to regain eccentric efficiency than concentric, but the eccentric strength is the more important for basic joint protection.

Accurate and efficient muscle function depends on your nervous system and your circulatory system. The flow of fluids into and out of muscles ensures that the muscles have sufficient nutrition to supply their energy needs, and that the waste products from muscle activity are removed efficiently. When you choose to perform a certain movement, your brain sends a signal through your nervous system to the nerve which controls the relevant muscle group. This process is called neuromuscular co-ordination. Some people are naturally better co-ordinated for certain types of movement than others, but if you want to improve a skilled movement

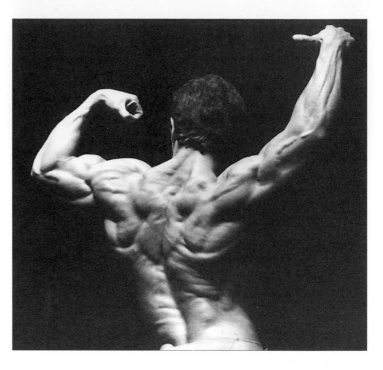

The complex muscles of the back

involving co-ordination and balance, you can generally do so through practice with appropriate guidance (feedback), at least up to a point.

In any kind of injury, or when pain from any cause affects a part of the body, the circulatory system is usually undermined, and resolving this is crucial both for tissue healing and for efficient muscle and joint function. In injury there is always disruption to the neuromuscular system, and you lose a certain amount of your normal co-ordination, depending on the severity of the pain and how long it lasts. Injury undermines the basic strength of the muscles around the damaged part by inhibiting their normal function. Around damaged spinal joints, the muscles often go into spasm (tightness, or unremitting slight contraction). All this has to be corrected for a return to full, efficient function.

Muscle groups acting on the spinal bones and related joints

The muscles which activate the different parts of the back and neck are arranged in a complicated format, because the joint formations and functions which they control are also complex. Around the pelvis are several muscle groups which create movements in the hips and the lower back. The front of the trunk is controlled by the large abdominal and pectoral muscles, while along the back itself and up into the neck are large and small muscles designed to stabilize and move the spinal joints.

The abdominal muscles which link the ribs to the front and sides of the pelvic basin have a variety of vital functions in relation to the trunk and spine. They contract when you cough, sneeze, pass faeces or urine, or lift a heavy weight. They act to bend the trunk into flexion against gravity, for instance when you are lying on your back and lift your head up or do sit-ups. They work eccentrically to control the movement of backward bending (extension) when you do this standing up. The abdominals are arranged so that they can work in a straight line, or into the twisting movements which allow you to turn to either side. They have a vital role in stabilizing the pelvis: if they are tight, they pull the pelvis into a backward tilt, and if they are weak they allow the pelvis to fall forwards in an increased forward tilt which exaggerates the arch in the low back (lumbar lordosis). Efficient abdominal muscles are essential elements for protecting the trunk and spine.

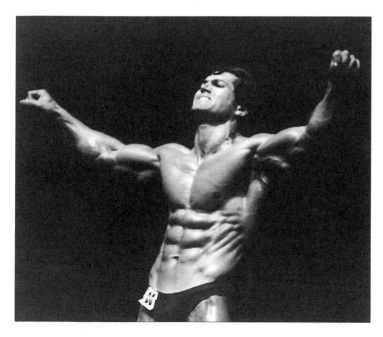

The muscles covering the front of the trunk, including the pectorals and abdominals

The back extensors (erector spinae) form a large sheet of muscle made up of distinct parts arranged in such a way from top to bottom that they can bend any part of the vertebral column backwards (into extension) against gravity, or control forward bending under the influence of gravity. It spreads out sideways from the spinous processes so that it controls all the interlinked joints of the vertebral column. You can feel the edges of the erector muscles as the strong, prominent muscles on either side of the spinous processes in the centre of the backbone.

The back extensor and multifidus muscles act together to raise the trunk and head upwards against gravity when you lie on your front. They start the same movement when you are standing up but, once started, backward bending is then mainly controlled by the eccentric action of the abdominals. When you bend forwards while standing up, the back extensors work eccentrically to control the movement, although when you are fully bent the extensor muscles relax, as the movement is controlled by the joint structures alone.

The low back muscles control the pelvis from behind: if they are tight, the pelvis tilts forwards and the curve in the low back is accentuated, while weakness has the opposite effect. The upper parts of the erector muscles control movements in the upper back (thoracic spine), neck and head. At each part of the spine, the muscles are arranged to achieve appropriate movements, such as twisting, bending, extending and side-bending. The degree of each movement in the different segments is controlled by the configuration of the joints and their controlling ligaments.

The transversospinalis is a complex arrangement of short, deep-seated muscles set out in the different regions of the vertebral column. The muscles consist of the semispinalis muscles, which lie in the upper back, neck and join on to the base of the skull, the rotatores which extend from the low back to the neck, and the multifidus muscle which goes all the way from the sacrum to the middle part of the neck. These muscles can bend the trunk backwards and sideways, or twist it, and they also act as postural muscles, helping to keep the trunk upright against gravity. Quadratus lumborum is a rectangular-shaped muscle which links the top of the iliac crest, the transverse processes at the sides of the vertebrae and the twelfth rib. It helps to extend the spine against a resistance, but its main functions are to bend the trunk sideways in conjunction with the other muscles which achieve this, and to stabilize the twelfth ('floating') rib as you breathe.

Latissimus dorsi extends right over the back and up to the front of the shoulder. It is attached to the iliac crest and sacrum at its lower part, to the lumbar and lower six thoracic spinous processes, spreading over the back of the ribs and across the tip of the shoulder blade (scapula), finally winding underneath the shoulder to its attachment point at the top of the arm-bone. The muscle forms the fold of flesh behind the armpit (axilla), together with another muscle, teres major, which comes away from the shoulder blade. Because it is such a large muscle, covering so many different parts of the back, it has several functions, including drawing the arm down towards the body into adduction, backwards into extension and inwards into medial rotation.

Latissimus dorsi contracts when you cough, sneeze or take a deep breath. Its main action is to draw the arm inwards and backwards against gravity or a resistance, as in crawl swimming. It works when you support your bodyweight on your hands, for instance doing the pommel horse discipline in male gymnastics, or simply lifting your body out of a chair using your hands and arms. Another function is to pull your body upwards through your arms in rock climbing or when you do 'chin-ups' to a bar (hanging by your arms and pulling your bodyweight up towards the bar). The nerves which control the muscle come out from the lower neck in the upper part of the spinal cord (technically C6, 7 and 8), so that the muscle can still function even when the spinal cord has been damaged or severed below that level. This can make it possible for someone who has suffered paralysis through spinal injury to use crutches for standing upright and moving about, even though the legs themselves cannot work.

The hip flexors, psoas major and iliacus (collectively known as iliopsoas), together with the longest muscle in the quadriceps group, rectus femoris, act to bring your thigh forwards at the hip against gravity, technically into flexion, for instance as you walk and run forwards. Iliopsoas also acts when you lift your trunk up from lying on your back. If the hip flexors are tight, they bend the hip (into flexion) and pull the pelvis into an increased forward tilt, which increases the arch of the low back (lumbar lordosis). If the muscles are tight on one side only, they may create a torsional effect on the sacroiliac joints on either side of the pelvis by pulling one side forwards relative to the other. If the hip flexors are weak, they may fail to hold the pelvis in normal balance, so the low back curve may be reduced or flattened slightly.

The hamstrings, which are attached to your seat bone (ischial tuberosity), act to lift the leg backwards, technically into extension, from the hip. As their lower attachments are below the knee at the top of the shin-bone (tibia) and the outer leg-bone (fibula), they also act to bend the knee. In sprinting, the hamstrings have to work through their full range, going from maximum stretch at full length to their shortest position, which is why sprinters so often suffer explosive hamstring injuries during races. As the hamstrings are attached to the back of the pelvis, they exert pressure against the bone. If the hamstrings on both sides are tight, they pull the pelvis into a backward tilt, flattening the arch of the low back (lumbar lordosis). If they are weak, they may allow the pelvis to tip forwards, accentuating the low back curve. If the hamstrings on one side are tight, while the other side is relatively weak, there may be an unbalancing torsional effect on the pelvis.

The main gluteal muscles, the gluteus maximus on either side, form the rounded contour of your bottom and move the thigh backwards from the bent position into extension, an important movement in cross-country skiing or when you drive off one foot in running or jumping. When you straighten your trunk up from standing bent over forwards, the gluteus maximus muscles activate to raise your upper body relative to your hips and legs.

On each side of the pelvis and hips are the hip abductor muscles (gluteus medius and minimus) which lift the legs sideways against gravity or a resistance when you are standing up or lying down. The hip abductors have an important role in stabilizing the pelvis during standing and walking. If you stand on one leg, the hip abductors on the side of the weightbearing (standing) leg work to hold the pelvis level, while the hip abductors on the other side activate to lift the leg off the floor. If the hip abductors on the weightbearing side are weak, the trunk tends to bend sideways to compensate, so that the other leg can be lifted off the floor. If the abductors are extremely weak, it is impossible to hold the pelvis level even by tilting the trunk sideways, so the hip on the unsupported side tends to drop downwards. This is called 'Trendelenberg's sign'.

Piriformis is another muscle which acts on the hip joint. It pulls the thigh out sideways (into abduction) when the hip is bent (flexed) and turns the thigh outwards (into lateral rotation) when the hip is extended. Piriformis lies close to the gluteus medius and its connection to structures of the sacroiliac joint gives it some influence in certain low back problems.

The main muscles controlling the upper back and shoulder girdle are trapezius, which links the neck and upper thoracic vertebrae to the collar-bone and shoulder blade (scapula), the rhomboids (major and minor), which connect the upper back to the shoulder blade, and levator scapulae, which lies between the neck and the shoulder blade. Trapezius consists of several parts: the upper part, with levator scapulae, lifts the top of the shoulder blade upwards, and also helps to bend the neck sideways when the shoulder is still; its outer part helps pull the shoulder blade forwards, together with the chest muscle serratus anterior; and the middle part combines with the rhomboids to draw the shoulder blades together. The rhomboids not only help pull the shoulder blades together, but in combination with levator scapulae and the chest muscle pectoralis minor they also pull the shoulder blade downwards.

Muscle imbalances which can affect the spinal joints

Relative tightness or weakness:
- between the muscles in front of and behind the trunk (anterior muscles = mainly the abdominals and pectorals posterior muscles = mainly the back extensors)
- between the muscles on either side of the trunk (mainly the side flexors which bend the trunk sideways and the rotators which twist the trunk)
- between muscles on either side of the midline in front of the trunk (across the abdomen and chest)
- between muscles on either side of the midline at the back (on either side of the backbone or spine)
- between individual muscles within a muscle group

If you habitually carry a heavy load on one shoulder, you are likely to over-develop the upper fibres of trapezius and the levator scapulae on that side. These muscles can also become tight for other reasons, such as viral infection or tension through stress and worry. If they do not function properly, the normal interaction with the shoulder muscles, deltoid and supraspinatus, is distorted. This tends to increase the muscle imbalance, and can contribute to neck pain.

Pectoralis major, which connects most of the ribs to the collar-bone, is the main muscle on the front of the chest, and it acts to draw your shoulder inwards. It co-ordinates with other muscles, notably latissimus dorsi, if you pull your bodyweight upwards using your arms, as in rock climbing. If the muscle is tight, it tends to pull the shoulders forwards, creating tension in the muscles across the upper back.

Serratus anterior and pectoralis minor link the ribs to the shoulder blade (scapula), and they are active in virtually all arm movements. They act together to bring the shoulder blade and arm forwards in reaching and pushing, so they are important for punching in boxing or tae kwon do, or throwing. Serratus anterior helps to stabilize the shoulder blade if the arm is moved to a small degree only, and it rotates the shoulder blade in order to allow the arm to be lifted fully sideways or upwards. If serratus anterior does not work properly, the inner edge of the shoulder blade tends to stick out. Arm movements are blocked, and if you try to force the arm to move, the shoulder blade juts out even further, forming a so-called 'winged scapula' .

Pain in the back and neck

4

If you have an accident, you expect to have pain, and you also expect the pain to go away with time. In this situation, the pain may be frightening, but the fear usually subsides with the acute pain. However, spinal pain, whatever its cause, can dominate your mind and take over your life, more so than pain in any other part of the body. There are many potentially worrying situations in different kinds of back and neck conditions. For example, pain can linger on long after an accident; pain can suddenly get much worse long after an accident; pain may occur during your customary physical activities in sport, recreation or work; and pain can occur for no apparent reason when you are 'doing nothing'.

It is normal to want the answers to the key questions arising in these situations: where has the pain come from? what damage has been done? how bad can it get? how long will it last? what can I do to make it go away? who can help me? Sometimes it is not easy to obtain quick and satisfactory responses to these questions, which is obviously frustrating.

Therefore it can be reassuring to know how pain relates to any damage that might have happened to the spinal structures. Pain and damage do not necessarily correlate in a logical fashion. Even if you are in a lot of pain, it does not necessarily mean that there is serious damage or disease.

In order to understand spinal pain, you need to know how it is caused, and how certain factors can make it worse even when there is no increase in tissue damage or trauma. If you understand the nature of spinal pain, you will be able to deal with it calmly and positively. This will in turn help you to respond to treatment and is vital for controlling and ultimately conquering the pain.

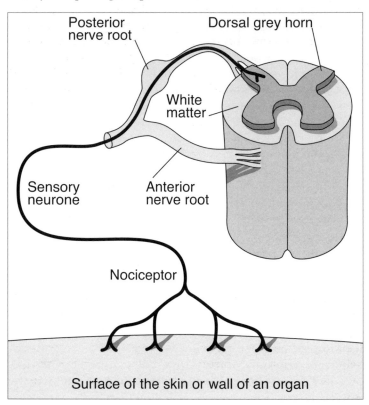

A pain nerve transmits signals from the damaged or inflamed tissue to the posterior horn of the spinal cord

WHAT THE PAIN MIGHT FEEL LIKE

Pain in any part of the back or neck can range from a feeling of stiffness and/or minor aching to the agonising, the excruciating and the unbearable. It might feel like superficial irritation, deep continuous burning, or acute shooting pain. It can be constant or intermittent. If constant, the pain can range from mild to severe. If it comes and goes, it might seem arbitrary and random or it can follow a recognizable pattern.

The pain might be localized to one spot, or spread diffusely over a wider area. It may be felt in the centre of an area in your back or neck, or it may feel concentrated to one side or the other of the spine. The pain may appear to affect different parts of the spine at different times, rather than one area consistently.

Pain radiating along the nerve pathways can form a tense line leading away from the spine. Symptoms referred through a nerve can vary, from a deep painful ache, a feeling similar to muscle cramp, to unpleasant tingling or numbness. Sometimes radiating nerve pain may be experienced without any pain in the associated area of the spine, so that the pain you feel does not seem to be connected with the back or neck. Headaches, similarly, can originate from neck problems, but they do not necessarily happen in conjunction with specific pain in the neck itself.

Your pain might vary according to your posture and activities. Immobility can ease or aggravate pain. Lying down may ease spinal pain, but in some cases it can intensify it. You may notice pain in bed overnight from lying still, or through twisting movements as you turn over. Lying in a certain position may relieve your pain, although this may prove to be only temporary. Sitting still may be comfortable or painful, and might vary according to the type of chair you are in. Standing still can similarly cause, increase or relieve spinal pain.

Certain movements may seem to relieve your pain, while others increase it. Walking about may help your pain if it is especially bad when you are standing still. But in other cases walking increases spinal pain. Similarly, some sports can help, others hinder. Sometimes, even if sports, movements or exercises relieve pain at the time, you may feel pain afterwards.

Normal body functions can cause an increase in spinal pain. Bowel movements can increase low back pain, which is also sometimes aggravated just by the action of sitting down on the toilet. Coughing and/or sneezing can be extremely painful, either in the spine itself or in the nerve pathways leading away from the problem area of the spine into the arm(s) or leg(s).

There may be a consistent daily pattern to your pain. For instance, you may notice that your back feels stiff or aches when you first wake up in the morning, and then it eases out as you get moving. Or the morning may be the best time, with little or no pain, but then the pain builds up during the day. The pain pattern can also vary day by day, or even hour by hour. Sometimes you may feel better for moving about and taking exercise, whereas at other times the same activities increase your pain. Sitting or lying down may be alternately helpful or painful. You may have morning stiffness or night pain during some phases, or relief through resting overnight at others.

WHAT PAIN CAN DO TO YOU

The apparently arbitrary nature of spinal pain makes it extremely difficult to live with. When it appears uncontrollable, it is all the more debilitating and frightening. It is vital to remember that there is usually a logical reason for any pain, and that in the vast majority of cases the pain can at least be controlled and alleviated, if not cured altogether.

When spinal pain is minor, you may just feel an irritating ache. If it is in your lower or upper back, it may make you shift around while you sit or stand. In your neck, it can make you feel you want to keep rubbing the sore area, or move your head to stretch and twist the joints a little in different directions.

More severe pain can affect the way you move and carry yourself. It can make you limp, or make you feel you want to twist yourself to avoid the pain when you are sitting down. Maybe you feel you cannot sit down at all, but prefer to stand or walk about. Even moderate pain can cause a distortion in your posture, pulling you into a bent or twisted position, or a combination of the two. Neck pain can make you hold your head to one side, avoid using your arm, or hitch your shoulder up towards the painful area. You may be conscious of stiffness in the painful area, causing restriction in your movements and making it impossible to turn, bend or twist in certain directions. Night pain may disrupt your sleep totally, or only at intervals, in which case you may still be able to get enough sleep for adequate rest overall.

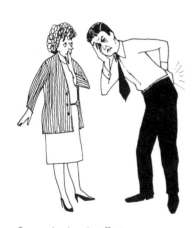

Severe back pain affects everyone around the patient

It is quite common to feel weakness in the affected spinal area, or in the body parts affected by radiating nerve pain, tingling or numbness. This happens for a number of reasons, for instance because of muscle injury and damage, or because the muscles are inhibited through malfunctioning in their nerve systems. This weakness makes it all the more tiring to try to maintain good upright posture against gravity, or to keep up normal everyday physical activities.

When spinal pain is at an excruciating level it is virtually impossible to think of anything else. The same applies if the pain you feel is radiating, with or without a direct connection to the spine itself. It is especially limiting if the pain affects the spine itself together with your arm(s), rib(s) or leg(s). You find your whole attention focused on the pain, which dominates all your everyday activities. If unremitting pain is present all or most of the time and it cannot be relieved by any normal painkilling methods, it inevitably affects you psychologically. Your sleep is also interrupted, so that you sleep fitfully, if at all.

The overall effect of excruciating pain emanating from the spine is usually totally debilitating, exhausting, depressing and frustrating. The same can also be said of any level of spinal pain, however dull or minor, which has lasted a long time, and which seems to be uncontrollable.

CHRONIC PAIN

When you have had a pain for a long time, it is described as chronic. This is not a term referring to the severity of the pain, although if you have a 'chronic pain syndrome' affecting any part of the spine it can be assumed that the pain is not only long-standing but also severe. A pain which has lasted for longer than six months can be described as chronic, and many chronic pain syndromes extend over several years.

During the prolonged period of pain, the victim has usually tried 'everything' to get rid of the problem, and may have had a wide variety of treatment procedures, including bedrest, drugs, physiotherapy, osteopathy, chiropractic, injections, surgery, Back Schools, Pain Clinics, acupuncture, reflexology and healing, to name but a few. It is also often the case that the chronic pain has disrupted every aspect of the victim's life. Employment of any kind may become impossible, as the chronic pain victim may not be able to sit or stand for any length of time, or carry even light bundles of papers, never mind lifting loads. Family life can be destroyed, marriages can break down, social activities may dwindle, and the victim becomes increasingly isolated and probably introspective about the apparently insoluble cycle of problems.

Not surprisingly, people in this situation often suffer from clinical depression as well. Their situation may be made worse by drug dependence. The addiction may be to painkillers or to the tranquillizers which are sometimes prescribed as muscle relaxants for spinal pain.

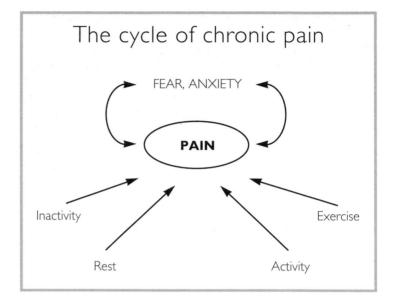

The cycle of chronic pain

FEAR, ANXIETY

PAIN

Inactivity

Rest

Activity

Exercise

CHILDREN'S PAIN

Spinal problems of all kinds become relatively common from the middle- to late-teen years onwards. Falls and accidents can cause back and neck pain in very young (pre-teen) children, but it is usually short-lived. It is unusual for children to suffer from the apparently spontaneous type of mechanical back pain which seems so common in middle-aged and older people. It is also rare for children to have referred nerve symptoms in the arms or legs.

It can be tempting to ignore or dismiss children's complaints of pain in the back or neck, in the hope that the child is exaggerating, or that the pain will disappear spontaneously. This approach is risky. Just in case this might be one of the very rare cases when something is seriously wrong, whether through physical injury, inflammation or disease, the child should be checked and screened. Otherwise there could be dangerous long-term consequences.

With children's pain, it is always better to err on the side of caution. Whenever a young child complains of any kind of pain affecting or relating to the spinal region, the responsible adult should try to help the child describe the pain and how it might have happened, so that the child's doctor has a clear picture of how it started and what might have caused it.

MECHANICAL CAUSES OF SPINAL PAIN

The majority of cases of pain in the back, neck or related areas are due to mechanical injuries, whether through accident or trauma, poor postural habits, or activities which disrupt normal function and create overload in the spinal joints. The amount of pain you feel does not always correlate with the severity of damage done to the injured structures. Actual tissue damage may be quite minor, yet the pain you feel can be appalling. Conversely, there may be objective signs of serious mechanical defects, for instance advanced joint degeneration which is obvious on X-rays, and yet comparatively little pain or limitation of function.

Injuries which involve a degree of traumatic shock can cause severe and long-lasting pain. A good example of this is whiplash injury from a car accident, where the victim's car is shunted from behind, thus throwing the victim's head and neck forcibly backwards. Even when there is no visible damage on X-ray initially or later, the patient's neck remains exquisitely tender and acutely painful for a long period, after which normal movement and function are recovered slowly but progressively. I always warn those of my patients who have suffered whiplash injury that the initial, frightening phase is likely to last for several weeks if not months, and that full recovery may take up to a year or even longer.

There are many different possible sources of spinal pain in different situations. It is not always possible to be precise about cause and effect in spinal problems, indeed in the majority of cases the processes remain a matter of guesswork. On the other hand, modern diagnostic techniques have offered new certainties in identifying specific tissue damage which can be responsible for different kinds of spinal pain. Some definitions have been established, although more research is needed because there is such a wide variety of potential causes of pain when one considers the whole range of spinal problems.

Mechanical problems which cause pain in the back and neck can be defined as resulting in three distinct types of pain: somatic pain, somatic referred pain and radicular pain.

Somatic pain

The technical term for pain which comes from one of the mechanical (skeletal) structures of the spine is somatic pain, which is sometimes also referred to as musculoskeletal pain. It can arise from any part of the bone, joint and muscular elements, but by definition does not involve nerve root compression or nerve disturbances (neurological abnormalities). However, it can give rise to referred pain (see p.71), which travels away from its source along nerve pathways, so that you feel the pain at some distance from the spine, with or without pain in the back or neck.

It is assumed that any structure which has a nerve supply is capable of being painful if it is damaged and diseased. Modern research methods have been able to demonstrate nerve distributions and the way in which pain is caused in great detail for many of the spinal structures. However, for some tissues, such as the vertebral bodies, epidural blood vessels, and structures in the upper back (thoracic spine), the studies are incomplete, and detailed pain analysis is still based on clinical observation, some guesswork and reasoned assumptions.

For a long time it was thought that the sacroiliac joints at the back of the pelvic basin could not be injured because they were effectively immobile. However, they are synovial joints, and it has gradually been accepted that they can become painful through mechanical injury, separately or together.

Throughout the whole spine, it is accepted that pain can arise from the facet joints (zygapophyseal joints), longitudinal ligaments, interspinous ligaments, intervertebral discs, dura mater, vertebral bodies and all the surrounding and supporting muscles. In the upper back (thoracic spine), pain may also arise from the joints between the vertebrae and the ribs (costotransverse joints). In the neck (cervical spine), the atlanto-occipital and atlanto-axial joints in themselves can also become painful, although their structure is very different from the other spinal joints.

In the intervertebral discs, the pain-sensitive nerves are confined to the outer part, the annulus fibrosus. This explains why it is possible to have severe degeneration of the central part of the disc (the nucleus pulposus) without any major pain. It is only when the outer part is damaged that pain arises from the disc. This happens if the annulus fibrosus itself is disrupted by a twisting (torsional) strain, overloaded through altered mechanics, degenerated because of degenerative processes in the rest of the disc, or impinged on by damaged material from the nucleus pulposus.

Somatic referred pain

Referred pain is pain which you perceive somewhere away from its actual source. When the referred pain relates to injury in the mechanical, musculoskeletal system, the usual technical term for it is somatic referred pain. This distinguishes this type of referred pain from the other types, which are related to the spinal nerve roots or disease, and are technically designated as radicular, visceral or vascular referred pain. Referred pain is often said to be caused by a 'trapped nerve', although this is a very imprecise expression which does not describe accurately what referred pain is or why it happens.

Any tissue which causes mechanical or somatic pain can also give rise to referred pain, so, for instance, referred pain can be triggered by injury or damage to ligaments, discs, the dura mater or the facet joints. The technical explanation for this seems to be that nerve impulses from the damaged tissue activate neurons (nerve cells) within the central nervous system which also receive messages from other parts of the body. This results in pain signals which seem to come from the other body parts, but without any signs of localized damage which might explain the pain.

Somatic referred pain generally seems to be a deep ache. It is often spread diffusely through the area of referral, so that it is hard to pinpoint exactly. Referred symptoms usually affect one side of the body only, but it is also possible to have pain radiating to both sides of the body simultaneously. From the sacroiliac joint, pain can be referred down the back of the thigh on the same side, usually stopping just above the knee. From the low back, somatic referred pain can be transmitted into one buttock or both, one leg or both, round into the groin on one or both sides, and sometimes into the abdominal region.

From the lower part of the upper back, pain can be referred downwards into the low back, and sometimes into the abdominal region. Pain from the rest of the upper back may be transmitted round the rib cage and into the chest wall, so you may feel pain behind your back or to the front of your chest. It can also be referred up into the neck and head, or up and round to the front of the shoulder and arm. Similar patterns of referred pain can develop from the neck too. Therefore referred pain in the head, shoulder, shoulder girdle, arm, and round the front or back of the chest wall (rib cage region) may as easily have its source in the neck as in the upper back.

Radicular pain

Problems in the vertebral column can cause disruption of the nerve roots, which is technically termed radicular or root pain. It gives rise to referred pain, and also to tingling sensations or 'pins and needles' (technically paraesthesiae), numbness or weakness in the areas which the particular nerves serve. These symptoms are called neurological signs, and any of them may occur in problems involving radicular pain. The symptoms may feel very similar to those caused by somatic referred pain. The difference is that in somatic referred pain the nerve roots are definitely not involved, so the mechanisms causing the symptoms are different. Somatic referred pain is described as being less well defined, and less sharp and searing in quality than radicular pain.

Apart from being referred to as 'trapped nerve syndrome' and lumped together with other types of referred pain in spinal problems, radicular referred pain is often defined as 'nerve root compression'. Modern research shows that the exact mechanisms by which nerve roots cause radicular pain are complicated. The symptoms may vary according to which specific parts of the nerve roots are injured through compressive pressure: the dorsal root ganglions can cause symptoms even if they have never been damaged before, whereas the nerve roots themselves are only likely to cause symptoms if they have been damaged previously. Any 'pins and needles' (paraesthesiae) may be caused by pressure on the blood vessels serving the damaged nerve root(s).

Radicular pain is generally accompanied by pain where the source is in the back or neck. It is generally agreed that nerve root disruption cannot cause spinal pain without also causing referred symptoms.

Compression on a particular nerve root normally leads to both sensation disturbance and muscle weakness in the pathway of the nerve, so that there is a distinct pattern to the symptoms which follows the anatomy of the nerve. Sciatica is a particular example of nerve root problem in which pain and symptoms are transmitted from the low back down the backs of the leg(s) along the pathway of the sciatic nerve. If the femoral nerve root is compressed, pain and neurological symptoms travel down the front of the thigh. In the upper back, nerve root compression can cause symptoms in a band round the rib cage, while in the neck the symptoms are usually felt down one side or the other of one arm, depending on the level at which the compression has occurred. Because of the anatomical structure of the uppermost vertebral joints, the atlanto-occipital and atlanto-axial joints, root compression is unlikely to occur, so it is considered that these problems only affect the neck from the third vertebra downwards.

HOW PAIN IS CAUSED

Pain happens when pain-transmitting (technically nociceptive) nerve endings are stimulated. There are basically two ways in which this happens: one is through chemical irritation, the other through mechanical irritation. In the former, it is thought that certain chemicals are released from damaged cells, and directly affect the pain nerve endings. This can happen when tissues have been affected by inflammatory diseases, and also as an after-effect of mechanical tissue damage. Mechanical irritation causes over-stretching of connective tissue, the normal fabric of all the mechanical body structures, which evidently puts pressure on the pain nerves, stimulating them to send out their pain signals.

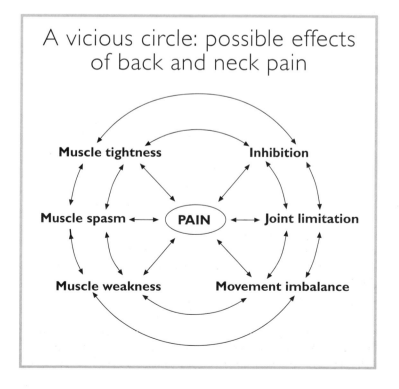

A vicious circle: possible effects of back and neck pain

Muscle tightness

Inhibition

Muscle spasm ←→ PAIN ←→ Joint limitation

Muscle weakness

Movement imbalance

ALTERNATIVE CAUSES OF SPINAL PAIN

Like most practitioners, I have treated many patients who have complained of apparently simple back or neck pain, but whose problems turn out not to be injuries at all, but to be due to other sources.

Tumours can cause searing pain in the spinal region. As malignant disease spreads through the body in the late stages, secondary growths can lodge in the lower back region or round the chest wall in the upper back. Sometimes this happens without causing particular pain, but if there is pain it can be horrifyingly intense. Fortunately, such cases are very rare, and very few people are likely to suffer from this type of spinal pain.

Much more common are cases of spinal pain relating to infections of various kinds. Many different viruses, infections or illnesses can give rise to aches and pains which might seem musculoskeletal, but which in fact are pain-causing in themselves. These conditions of apparent spinal pain may arise through infections introduced into the victim's body by the various pathways that viruses and bacteria can take. Kidney infections, for instance, can be a direct cause of acute back pain, while chest infections like pleurisy can cause pain in the upper back or in the trapezius muscle leading up one side of the neck. Gynaecological problems or hormonal changes can also cause low back pain in females. Sometimes an inexplicable backache is the first sign of pregnancy.

Some hereditary or familial inflammatory conditions can also cause symptoms affecting the spine, so there may be a family history in which a parent or other relative has had similar problems. A few conditions which can cause spinal symptoms are not yet properly understood, so we do not know what causes them.

Sometimes injury problems co-exist alongside symptoms relating to a virus or an infection, but in other cases the illness alone is responsible for the pain. Even when the pain is solely due to illness, inflammatory disease or infection, the patient is usually quite convinced that it must be due to some injury, although no obvious trauma has happened to explain it. The pain may feel exactly the same as mechanically caused spinal pain which might affect the muscles, ligaments, discs or bones. To confuse the issue further, there may also be mechanical symptoms such as muscle spasm over the painful area, so that the practitioner may not realize immediately that the problem is not purely mechanical.

BACKGROUND FACTORS IN SPINAL PAIN

Where the level of pain is disproportionately severe in relatively minor mechanical problems, several different background factors may play a part. Sometimes, such factors can be the dominant cause in a spinal problem, but more often they simply add to the pain you feel. They can also contribute to pain caused by inflammatory conditions, diseases or viral infections.

Fear, depression and stress

Pain relating to spinal problems can be very frightening, especially if it is out of all proportion to any injury you have suffered. The situation is even worse if you have not suffered an injury at all, and the pain seems to come from 'out of the blue'. Fear and stress both intensify the pain you feel. All too often, you can find yourself caught in a vicious circle where relatively minor back or neck problems cause increasingly savage pain, because your awareness of the pain has been magnified by your fear of it.

Because fear heightens your perception of pain, the more frightened you are, the more you feel the hurt. If you are anxious that you might have something seriously wrong with you, or frightened about your injury and what damage might have occurred, or indeed if you are worrying about some other, quite separate, trouble in your life, you are likely to focus on the pain more than it deserves, and this in turn magnifies it, increasing your level of anxiety. Your sensitivity and pain are therefore exacerbated in an ever-worsening spiral.

If you are really low emotionally, to the extent of being clinically depressed, you tend to focus on your problems and pain in a negative way, without any positive hope that things are going to improve. This inevitably makes your perception of pain greater, increases your tension and apprehension, and at the same time reduces your ability to work out what to do to solve your problems. Your muscle tone drops when you are clinically depressed, so that your muscles effectively become weakened and feel 'flabby'. If you try to take exercise or perform physical tasks, you notice how difficult you find the effort, and how quickly you become unreasonably tired.

The reduction of muscle tone means that your trunk muscles cannot provide a normal level of stability and protection for your spinal joints, so they are more susceptible to damage.

I had treated a certain patient, S., some years previously for back pain, and since then he had been working out regularly doing a fitness programme using weights and circuit training. He had maintained a good level of fitness, but one day he came to see me, complaining of an acute recurrence of quite severe back pain. As I examined him, I was perturbed to find that his spinal muscles felt extremely 'flabby' (low-tone), despite the fact that he had been training consistently, and had not been ill or injured. After a little gentle probing, S. quietly began to cry, and then revealed that he was suffering extreme emotional stress due to marital problems. I suggested that he should consult a psychologist, which he did. Counselling helped him to recover to some extent, and his back pain eased almost instantly. He was then able to continue his physical training without setbacks, and this was an important element in overcoming remaining emotional problems.

Food intolerance

When you are worried, whether specifically about your back problem or generally about life's stresses, you may become more susceptible to food intolerance reactions. This means that certain foods or drinks, or certain dietary combinations, may cause irritation in your vulnerable joints.

In my experience, it is rare for food intolerance actually to cause spinal pain, although I have seen very many cases of food intolerance in the hands, knees, feet and elbows which are the joints most commonly affected by food intolerance. The example of one of my patients, K., shows how food intolerance can be implicated in spinal problems. This case also illustrates how difficult it can be to identify the trigger substance if it is something which you believe is beyond suspicion.

K. began to suffer from neck pain, coupled with headaches and radiating pain down his left arm, which he associated with running. He was keen on keeping fit, and he enjoyed swimming and working out on a rowing ergometer. When I first examined K., it was clear that his pain pattern was unusual, and that there was an underlying and probably obscure cause for the symptoms. There did not seem to be any hint of disease, but he was screened by the consultant rheumatologist just in case, and because he needed reassurance that he was not suffering from some serious condition. Manual therapy was given, and after about three weeks K. was working out in my rehabilitation gymnasium using the Norsk equipment once or twice a week over several weeks. Generally, he was symptom-free during this period, but he occasionally relapsed, for no obvious reason, and when he did so he became extremely anxious about his state of health.

Eventually K. realized that his neck pain and headaches were directly linked to drinking a certain brand of carbonated water: this had been the only element of his diet which he had not questioned during several months of monitoring his pain pattern. He confirmed his suspicion by avoiding the water for some days, during which he was pain-free, and then drinking it again. He reported that the symptoms returned within about an hour every time he drank that particular water. The discovery enabled him to control his problem, and K. learned to be very vigilant about his food and drink intake and any reactions resulting from it.

More commonly, food intolerance simply plays a subsidiary role in aggravating spinal pain which has come on through other causes. It can play a particularly large part in conditions where female hormonal change is also a factor, such as the apparently spontaneous 'frozen shoulder' which can be linked to the menopause (see p.80).

Food intolerance: symptoms

- headache
- pain in one or more joints
- stiffness in one or more joints
- skin redness
- 'burning' sensation in the skin or joint(s)

Anyone can develop an intolerance to any kind of foodstuff, even to something eaten regularly over a long time. Certain foods and drinks are especially likely to cause reactions, including citric fruits such as oranges and lemons, juices, chocolate, cheese, alcohol and fizzy drinks. Identifying food intolerance is a matter of detective work. If you notice that there is an increase in pain within an hour or two of eating or

Food intolerance: causes and effects

Potentially irritant foods include:
citrus fruits, tomatoes, juices, spicy foods, pork, shellfish, cereals, eggs, cow's milk, fizzy drinks, alcoholic drinks, tea, coffee, chocolate, preservatives, colouring

Symptoms usually appear within an hour or two of eating and drinking the irritant, but in the case of wheat the reaction can take a couple of days to show up.

drinking a particular substance, you should try leaving it out for a while, and see if that makes any difference to your pain. If you suspect that you might be intolerant to wheat, you should try to go for about four days at a time without eating bread or other wheat products, as it can take up to a couple of days for a reaction to wheat to show up.

Even if you do not identify food and drink as a factor in your pain, it is always a wise precaution to make sure that you eat regular meals three times a day, taking in a wide variety of foods including plenty of green vegetables, and that you drink a lot of plain water throughout each day. You should avoid, or at least reduce, coffee, tea or alcohol. You should certainly cut out 'junk' foods, chocolate and fizzy drinks. It is rash to assume that your diet is 'healthy' and that therefore food intolerance cannot happen to you. Even supposedly 'healthy' foods can cause reactions.

Food intolerance: prevention

- Avoid potentially irritating food or drinks
- Cut down on tea, coffee and alcohol
- Eat regular, well-balanced meals
- Eat plenty of green vegetables
- Vary your diet as much as possible
- Avoid stress and fatigue
- Drink plenty of plain water all day, every day

An inadequate diet can also complicate some spinal problems: for instance, vitamin B12 deficiency can cause tingling sensations in the hands, and this can seem identical to the tingling produced by nerve disruption in certain types of neck problem. Sometimes the patient has both referred symptoms from the neck and the tingling due to the vitamin deficiency.

Female hormones

Hormonal changes in females can have an impact on spinal pain. With the onset of her periods (technically menarche), a girl might notice a degree of backache just before she is 'due' each month. Sometimes this may be only very slight, at other times it may seem quite bad, but it tends to pass shortly after the period has started.

In the late teens, when the hip and pelvic bones are going through their final development phase, roughly between the ages of 17 and 19, the low back may seem especially vulnerable to strain just before each period. This may be because the ligaments of the pelvic joints alter their consistency premenstrually.

I have treated many cases of this kind of back problem in young female sports players. Typically, the back 'goes' when the athlete does a particular routine involving some shearing of the sacroiliac joints, such as hill- or bend-running. Young female tennis players may experience the same thing as a result of a practice session or match, when the twisting motion for stroke production suddenly becomes overtaxing for the sacroiliac joints. The activity is usually not particularly demanding for the player, and would not be expected to cause problems in the normal way. The injury is not necessarily related to cold or fatigue, as the strain can happen at any stage of the session. Once it has happened, it is usually acutely painful, but can be expected to settle quickly with gentle treatment, rest from physical activities for a couple of days, and remedial exercises.

The contraceptive pill

The contraceptive pill usually helps to reduce backache associated with premenstrual tension or painfully heavy periods (dysmenorrhoea). However, arguably, unless it is being used for its primary contraceptive purpose, it should probably not be used to control menstruation-linked backache. There are other possible ways of doing this which avoid the potential health risks which may be associated with the pill.

After childbirth, the mother must be guided by her doctor or gynaecologist before going back on to the pill. One young mother I treated suffered excruciating and apparently unexplained 'agony' in her upper back (thoracic spine) which dragged on for some weeks. Fitness training, remedial exercises and treatment neither relieved nor aggravated her pain. After careful consideration, we realized that her pain had started when she began to take the pill again. She had done this very early, against her doctor's advice, while she was still breastfeeding her baby. Within days of stopping taking the pill, the upper back pain had gone. When this mother gave birth to a second very healthy baby nearly three years later, she avoided making the same mistake, and allowed plenty of time before thinking of taking the pill again.

Any kind of hormone changes, such as going on to or coming off the contraceptive pill, or changing the particular brand of pill you use, can cause or influence backache. It is therefore important to allow time for adjustment if you make any such changes. In the transition phase, you may also need to alter your diet to create greater variety, while maintaining healthy and regular eating habits.

The menopause

In later life, the menopause brings with it various profound body changes in females. The symptoms of the menopause vary between individuals: some women scarcely notice the change, whereas others can suffer quite badly from effects such as headaches, vision disturbance, joint pains, mood swings and sometimes depression. The most potentially damaging effect of this phase of hormonal change is the increased risk of osteoporosis, or 'brittle bones' (see p.147). Osteoporosis is usually hereditary, but it can be linked to a poor diet and other factors.

One relatively common problem among female patients which tends to coincide with the menopause (although it can also happen earlier or later) is the so-called 'spontaneous frozen shoulder'. One shoulder becomes extremely painful, either suddenly or in gradual stages, and then seizes up so that it is virtually impossible to move in any direction. Untreated, or inadequately treated, the problem drags on for up to two years or more before it resolves itself apparently spontaneously. It can happen in either shoulder, and it is not uncommon for each shoulder to be affected in turn, although it is extremely rare for both shoulders to suffer at once.

Treatment has to be directed at the upper back (thoracic spine), and the practitioner must avoid irritating the shoulder itself in any way until the acute phase of inflammation has passed. In my experience, this problem is avoidable if the upper back is treated as soon as the first slight sign of shoulder pain appears, and if the patient alters her diet and does appropriate remedial exercises.

Hormone Replacement Therapy

Hormone Replacement Therapy (HRT) is commonly prescribed to reduce the risk of osteoporosis, and it is said to carry other benefits as well, such as reducing joint problems and the risk of heart disease. If it is prescribed accurately, it certainly helps to minimize the negative effects of the menopause, such as low moods and irritability. HRT is essential if there is a history of osteoporosis in the family, or if scanning shows that the patient is vulnerable to 'brittle bones'. It is not prescribed if there are contra-indications such as a history of malignant disease (cancer).

It is probably true to say that HRT should not be taken routinely just because a woman has reached middle age. Firstly, it does not suit all women, and some feel quite uncomfortable taking it. Secondly, not all women need it, as many pass through the menopause without feeling any particular ill-effects from it. Thirdly, in my clinical experience, it is possible that HRT can produce some uncomfortable and undesired side effects. I have seen cases where aching or sometimes even acute pain in the sacroiliac joint has coincided with placing the HRT patch close to that joint, and where the ache or pain disappear when the patch is applied further away on the thigh. Similarly, even in cases when the HRT has been taken orally, low back pain has sometimes occurred.

A 69-year-old patient, A., had fallen and injured her right shoulder. Osteopathic treatment five weeks after the trauma had resulted in much worse shoulder pain, with the result that she could hardly move her arm. She had been taking HRT for many years with her general practitioner's encouragement. When I started to treat her and after discussion with her GP, we decided that she should stop taking the HRT. Within about a week, A.'s shoulder pain was much better. Treatment was directed at the upper back (thoracic spine) at first, and the patient had to alter her diet, as she occasionally suffered from obvious food intolerance reactions. Within six weeks it was possible to start manipulating the shoulder itself, and A. was able to carry light loads in her right hand. Progress was then steady, and four months after the start of treatment the patient had recovered a good range of movement and was able to use the right arm functionally again.

It is obviously important to discuss the pros and cons of taking any kind of hormonal drug with your doctor or specialist, and to monitor your reactions to any new drug, so that changes can be made immediately if necessary. It is also helpful to remember that hormonal changes may make you more sensitive to irritation through food and drink, so you should try to become aware of any food intolerance reactions, and adjust your diet to prevent them.

Pregnancy and childrearing

Pregnancy 'loosens' the ligaments in the pelvic joints, as they have to become increasingly lax to allow for the development and ultimate delivery of the baby. Backache during pregnancy is extremely common, which makes it very important to do appropriate exercises throughout the pregnancy, preferably under guidance from a specialist obstetric chartered physiotherapist. Sometimes the first sign of a pregnancy is a sudden, unexplained backache, a month or two after conception. This usually eases spontaneously as the pregnancy becomes established.

Childbirth itself can give rise to subsequent back pain for a variety of reasons. In a natural birth, a big baby can cause over-stretching of the pelvic ligaments. When pain relief through a total epidural injection is given, the mother loses any sensation in the pelvis and legs for the duration that the epidural lasts, so it is vital for the carers and nurses attending the mother to maintain her hips and legs in the correct position throughout the birth. If the legs are allowed to flop at an awkward angle, there may be dangerous pressure through the hips into the pelvic joints. The so-called 'mobile' epidural affords pain relief, but allows the mother greater control over her movements. However it has to be very expertly administered: I have known cases of back problems and radiating nerve pain which apparently arose as a result of imperfectly given mobile epidural injections.

Following childbirth, the mother has to cope with the after-effects of the trauma of labour, plus the need to lift and handle the baby who, in normal circumstances, is rapidly increasing in size and weight day by day. During the period of breastfeeding, it is fairly common for the mother to experience joint pains especially in the small joints of the fingers. This is usually only temporary, passing when breastfeeding has finished, but it can be quite unpleasant. Back pain during the early phase of caring for a baby is usually mechanical, caused by having to lift, carry and transfer the baby at an awkward angle. There is more risk to the back if the mother has a heavy pram, or a low baby cot or bath which forces her to lean over while holding the baby.

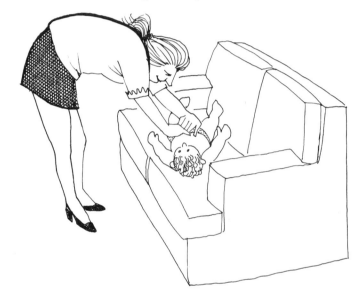

Awkward bending is a hazard for the new mother

PAIN PATTERNS: WHAT THEY MEAN

One of the hardest things for patients to understand about back pain is just how imprecise it can be in relation to its cause. For several reasons, your practitioner cannot tell what is causing your pain and how it should be treated simply by knowing where you are feeling it. Firstly, where you perceive your pain may not necessarily be the actual place from which the pain originates. Secondly, nerve distributions are very imprecise, and variable from person to person. Referred pain is especially difficult to track down to one region in the spine, even if it follows a well-defined course. Thirdly, your pain may in fact have several different sources, rather than just one, and it may involve more than one pain-causing mechanism.

All of this makes it extremely important for you to avoid any attempt at self-diagnosis. You should try to become aware of when and how your pain(s) and any other symptoms happen, without drawing any conclusions from them.

The next chapter tells you how to set about dealing with your problem according to your situation.

Coping with back and neck pain

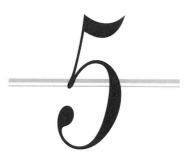

FIRST AID

Most back and neck injuries, however painful, do not involve major damage to vital structures. First aid is a matter of pain management until the victim can see a qualified practitioner for checks and treatment. However, everyone involved in sport has to remember that major traumatic injuries affecting the spinal joints carry the risk of causing paralysis, if the injury is severe enough to damage the spinal cord. This danger exists in sports like show jumping, gymnastics and acrobatics, and has to be minimized where possible by good safety practices.

Damage to the spinal cord usually happens if the vertebral bones are fractured, but it can also happen without any bone injury. A bad injury which disrupts the top of the neck can even kill the victim. From the first-aid point of view, it is important to know exactly what has happened to the victim in the accident, in order to understand what effect the injury might have had on vital structures in the back or neck. When dealing with possible spinal injuries, the first aider's priorities are to save life, and to avoid making the situation worse by doing the wrong thing.

Hasty actions can lead to tragic mistakes. A freak accident happened during a professional basketball game in 1995. A player jumped up to score a goal, and hit his head hard on a hoarding which was incorrectly mounted too close to the playing area. He immediately lost all feeling in his body, and collapsed on to the floor. Team mates and others in the vicinity thought he was fooling around and tried to lift him up, despite his pleas not to be moved. Paramedics arrived, but mistakenly thought he needed resuscitation, even though he was still breathing, so they manhandled the player in order to do mouth-to-mouth breathing.

The player's condition was undoubtedly made worse by the lack of proper care immediately after the accident. He was operated on, but not successfully, and was left paralysed in all four limbs (quadriplegic). He then had to face the long, slow journey through intensive rehabilitation to regain some function in his arms which might give him a degree of independent life, such as the ability to feed himself. The accident alone was enough of a personal tragedy. The mistakes made by people at the time added to the bitter experience with which the player had to come to terms, giving him more cause for grief, anger and frustration. Bitterness is rarely a positive motivator psychologically.

The most urgent action to take when someone has had any severe injury affecting the head, neck or back is to call the emergency services. Unless life-saving measures are needed, non-medically qualified first-aiders should not rush to intervene and treat the victim. If it is necessary to move the victim, for instance a jockey who has fallen in the middle of the racecourse, a special stretcher should be used if possible to avoid unnecessary movement in the spinal joints, and several people should help, provided they all know how to lift and transfer the suspected spinally injured patient correctly. Speed of action is important, but avoiding over-hasty and clumsy movements is even more so.

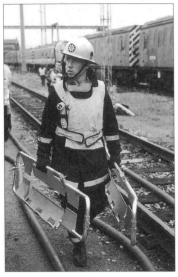

A 'scoop' stretcher, specially designed for lifting a spinally injured patient without causing further damage

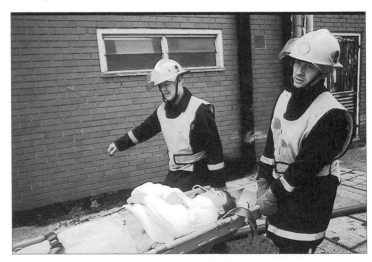

Any kind of direct force against the head can cause concussion or brain contusion. This is an obvious danger in boxing and lacrosse, and is a good reason why protective headgear should be worn in all situations where the head could be hit, such as contact sports, tae kwon do, American football, cricket (batting and wicket keeping), horse riding, roller skating, stock car racing, motorbiking and cycling. Similar effects can happen indirectly, if the neck is shaken very violently or hit. If the victim is at all disorientated, he or she must be taken to hospital for checks and observation. Even if hospital treatment is not necessary, the victim should not be allowed to be alone overnight. Both victim and carers should be ready to return to hospital quickly if further symptoms develop later, such as severe headache or neck pain.

First aid should always be kept as simple as possible. Even if an accident has happened which does not seem to have been very dramatic or dangerous, caution should always prevail if the back or neck may have been involved, especially in the case of a young patient. For instance, if a young player complains that his neck has been jarred during a rugby game at school, the teacher or coach should not allow him to play on, but insist the player rests. To support the neck in the absence of a supportive cervical collar, a folded newspaper can be wrapped round, covered and held in place by a scarf. If there is the slightest hint that the player has been concussed, he should be taken to hospital immediately for a check-up and perhaps observation overnight. Even if he seems all right, the child's parents should be informed that he has taken a knock, so that they know to take him to hospital immediately if he develops any major symptoms such as vomiting or headache overnight, or to refer to their general practitioner if the child develops subsequent neck pain.

On no account should manipulation techniques or massage be applied as first-aid procedures by non-qualified personnel such as sports coaches. The chances of making a dangerous mistake when dealing with spinal injuries are simply too high.

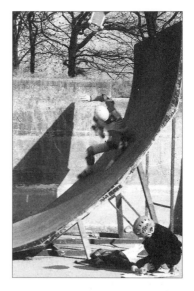

Protective headgear is a must in any sport which might cause a direct blow to the skull (especially in the young)

SELF-HELP MEASURES

If you have never had acute back or neck pain before, the first experience can be quite frightening. You must try to keep calm and control the pain until you can see a casualty doctor or your practitioner for help and advice. If you are prescribed pain-relieving or anti-inflammatory drugs or homoeopathic remedies, you should take the medicine in accordance with the instructions given. If you are not clear about how the medicine should be taken, or if you are not satisfied that it is doing you good, you must discuss your doubts with the practitioner who has prescribed it. Even if you find that medicines relieve your pain completely, be careful not to assume that they have also cured your problem. Overdoing physical activities while your pain is artificially controlled by drugs can cause a bad adverse reaction afterwards. You can only assume your problem has gone when you have had several clear days without pain or painkillers.

Rest

Finding a comfortable position to rest in when you have acute back or neck pain is often extremely difficult. Pain may dictate the choice to a certain extent. If sitting and standing are painful, you may be more comfortable lying down or walking around. Lying down is not necessarily comfortable in every case. However, it does ease the pressure on the spinal discs and joints, so it is probably the safest position to be in for episodes of sudden acute spinal pain. It is important to lie straight. If you lie on your back, keep your knees bent, or support them so that your hips and knees are at right angles to your trunk. If you lie on your front, you may find it more comfortable to support your hips and perhaps your chest on a pillow. Sometimes another pillow under your shins helps you to relax more fully. Lying on your side, it is vital not to twist yourself around or prop your head up on one arm. You should use pillows to support your head, chest, and your uppermost arm and leg.

Rest is the most sensible answer to acute and severe pain, so you should try to rest in as comfortable a position as you can find, until you receive appropriate treatment, or the pain eases. If you absolutely *have* to go to work, low back pain may be relieved by using an elastic corset for support. At the very least, the corset reminds you to sit and stand straight, and it may ease the pressure on your back to some degree. Neck pain may be eased by a soft or rigid collar, depending on how much the neck needs to be immobilized in order to be comfortable. However, you should not drive if you need to wear a support collar, as it restricts your neck movements to some degree, and so invalidates your motor insurance.

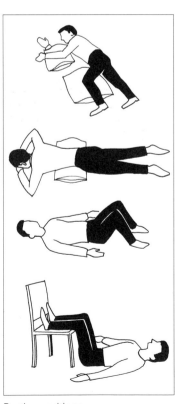

Resting positions

Soft and elastic supports do not cause weakness in your muscles, as you can still achieve slight joint movement and muscle activity while you wear them. Any support may become hot, or feel too restrictive after a while, especially during hot weather or in a warm environment, so you should then remove it for a period, taking care to maintain good posture at all times. If the support does relieve your pain significantly, you can wear it overnight as well as during the day, if it helps you to sleep better.

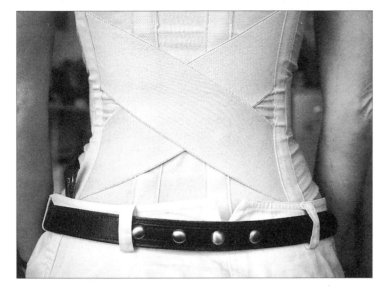

An elastic corset: in the recovery phases this belt is pliable enough to be worn for activities like tennis or gardening

Posture and pain control

Sitting is usually uncomfortable when there is pain in the back or neck. If you have to sit, you should use a high, well-shaped chair, and avoid sitting still for long periods. Sitting in a car seat can be extremely painful. If you have to make a car journey as a passenger and you have acute pain in your back or neck, try to lie down across the back seat with a pillow under your head and your knees bent. If you have to drive, make sure that you adjust your seat to achieve the best support you can manage, keeping your whole spine straight and your head supported. On a long journey, you should try to stop at frequent intervals so that you can walk around and stretch yourself out a little.

When you have to change positions after being still, try to get your joints moving first. Before you stand up after sitting down, gently arch your back, straighten your spine and lift your head up, then let your spine relax gently backwards. Do this a few times. It may also help if you do a few movements with your arms and legs as well. You have to bend forwards from the hips in order to get out of the chair, and it may be easiest if you push yourself up using your arms. When you have to get out of bed, try to do gentle arm and leg exercises, and arching and relaxing movements for your spine lying down. One way to get up is to lie close to the side of the bed, bend your knees to right angles, turn on to your side, and then push your trunk upwards with your hands while you let your legs down over the side of the bed. Sit on the side of the bed for a few moments, to avoid dizziness when you stand up. As changing your position can be one of the most painful aspects of back or neck pain, you may have to experiment to find out which way is easiest and least painful for your particular problem.

If you have to stand or walk in your job or for other reasons, you should wear well-fitting shoes with a slight heel, rather than very flat or high-heeled shoes. The soles should preferably be rubber and resilient. Cushioning insoles can help to reduce jarring, especially if the outer soles of your shoes are hard.

Ice and warm baths

For an acute injury which causes pain and muscle tightness (spasm), ice is usually helpful for reducing the discomfort. You can apply the ice by wrapping ice cubes in a damp cloth or flannel and placing it over the painful area for a few minutes. An alternative method of applying ice is for someone to rub an ice cube gently over the painful area for about one minute. You can also use ice packs, but take care to protect the skin with olive or baby oil, or a damp flannel. If you apply the ice for a short time only, you can repeat the treatment at frequent intervals without the risk of skin damage. The ice is easiest to apply if you can lie comfortably on your stomach, but if you find it better to lie on your back you can still make your ice pack or ice flannel very thin and place it under the painful area so that you lie on it. The effect of the ice is to reduce the sensitivity of your pain nerves, relieve muscle spasm to some extent, and stimulate the blood flow through the damaged or painful area.

Warm baths can also help to relieve spinal pain. You can relax in the warm water, and the overall effect is to stimulate the blood flow through your body, making it possible for you to move a little more easily. Water jets or a jacuzzi system in the bath can be very soothing. If your back problem makes it difficult for you to climb into the bath, you may still be able to manage by using a high bath seat to get over the water, and then a slightly lower one to lever yourself down into the water. Otherwise, a warm shower may help, especially for neck pain, when you can train the shower head against the painful side.

Even in the later stages of back or neck pain, the same measures can help to control and alleviate your pain. If your pain is intermittent, do not make the mistake of assuming that you are fully cured just because your pain has stopped temporarily. You need to go on looking after your back or neck until such time as you can perform all normal movements and activities without pain. Usually this means that you need to work through a progressive rehabilitation programme over a space of several weeks before you can be sure that you have regained full joint and muscle function.

Pain Control: Don'ts

- Don't try to ease pain by standing, sitting or lying crookedly
- Don't keep testing movements to find your pain
- Don't do things that are likely to cause pain
- Never do things you *know* will cause pain
- Don't resume normal activities until you have recovered fully

DIARY RECORD

Being able to describe the pain and its pattern accurately helps your practitioner to reach sensible conclusions as to what might be causing your problem, and how it should be treated. It is therefore both useful and important to keep a daily record of your pain, diet and activities, and any relevant background factors. When you feel pain, you should write down what kind of pain it was, what time it occurred and what you were doing at the time. If you have pain most of the time, you should take note of any periods when it gets worse, eases or disappears.

Your diary should provide a general outline of your normal daily activities in relation to your pain, and also any changes in your routine, such as home decorating or gardening. Your general health is also part of the picture, so you should record any medicines you have had to take for any reason, any illnesses or infections, and whether you have felt run down or especially tired. For females, it is important to note whether your pain changes in relation to your menstrual cycle, or other hormonal changes such as pregnancy, childbirth, the menopause or taking Hormone Replacement Therapy (HRT).

Pain Control: Do's

- Do rest during an acute episode of back or neck pain
- Do use pain-relieving techniques as recommended
- Do work out possible causes of your pain
- Do use protective supports if so advised
- Do use special seats, cushions or pillows as advised
- Do follow your practitioner's advice to the letter

Practitioners and treatment methods

6

WHERE TO START?

Anyone who suffers from a back or neck problem can come up against two linked difficulties, the first of identifying what the problem might be, and the second of knowing which practitioner to apply to for treatment. Self-diagnosis is impossible in spinal problems, so everything depends on finding the right practitioner to work out what is wrong and what to do about it.

In most countries, if you have any kind of physical or medical problem you go first to your general practitioner or family doctor. You may receive advice, medication, or referral for investigations or specialist treatment, as appropriate. For many types of complaint, the process is fairly straightforward. With back and neck pain, however, it is not necessarily clear at first sight whether the problem could be an arthritic condition, disease, or a mechanical derangement or injury. Even if the problem is mechanical, it may be doubtful whether specialist investigations are needed, or whether physical treatment is the right approach.

The problem is made worse by the fact that there are so many professional practitioners who are capable of giving physical treatment for spinal problems, so the general practitioner has to decide, for instance, between a physiotherapist, osteopath or chiropractor. These professions are usually classified as 'paramedical', although doctors may practise within them, particularly in the field of medical osteopathy. In the United States chiropractors have the title 'doctors' although their qualification is separate from the more standard medical training. The choice may appear to be arbitrary. A lot depends on the general practitioner's level of knowledge about spinal problems, his or her contact with different kinds of appropriate practitioner, and the availability of relevant professionals. Although many general practitioners limit their treatment to pain relief through drugs, some do physical treatments including manipulations, which can remove the need for further referral.

In fact, many back sufferers do not attend the general practitioner in the first instance, but go straight to a 'para-medical' practitioner. How the practitioner is chosen may be more a matter of luck than judgement. The worst way to find someone to treat you is to choose on the basis of assuming that what is wrong with you is the same problem that some-one you know had, and therefore the person who helped your acquaintance must be able to help you.

The sensible way to find an appropriate practitioner is to ask your general practitioner for help in the first instance.

DIAGNOSIS, ASSESSMENT AND TREATMENT

Successful treatment for spinal problems depends on many factors. The essential starting point is identifying your problem. This is done in two ways: firstly through the history and physical examination. This means that the practitioner pieces together the details of how your problem started and developed, and then assesses your condition through move-ment tests and by feeling the tissues. Secondly, investigations can be done, including blood tests, X-rays, myelograms and scans. In most cases of back and neck pain, the problem analysis is done on the basis of the physical assessment. Investigations are usually reserved for very severe problems, or if there is a special reason for doing them.

You may be disappointed if your practitioner gives you a seemingly vague definition of your problem. Generalized diagnoses such as 'disc problem', 'fibrositis' or 'lumbago' are made in order to be reassuring, even though they neither add to your understanding of your problem, nor prove that your practitioner knows what is wrong with you. There is no point in your practitioner inventing complicated hypotheses to show how clever he or she is, in situations when it is not possible to be absolutely precise.

Your only real guide to the accuracy of your practitioner's

assessment is the progress you make in recovering from your problem.

PRACTITIONERS

There are very many systems of treatment for back and neck problems, and there are different kinds of well-qualified practitioner who can treat spinal problems. There are also many low-qualified or even unqualified people who claim that they can treat spinal problems effectively. The treatment applied for any given problem is a matter of individual choice by the practitioner. The same practitioner may treat the same problem in different people using different techniques. Different practitioners will almost certainly use varying techniques and treatment modalities for dealing with the same type of problem in patients. Even within the same profession, treatment methods and techniques applied by each practitioner are extremely unlikely to be identical.

When choosing a practitioner, the minimum requirements are that the person should have a recognized professional qualification, and should be covered under professional indemnity insurance. Insurance against liability is important, just in case your treatment should go disastrously wrong and actually cause you harm. Although such cases are very rare, it is as well to know that you would be entitled to compensation if it were to happen.

What to expect from your practitioner

- Detailed questions and full physical assessment
- Explanation of what might be wrong
- Description of treatment techniques to be applied
- Statement of treatment aims
- Advice on correct posture
- Prescription of self-help measures
- Progressive rehabilitation exercise programme
- Reassessment at each treatment session
- Change of treatment techniques if unsuccessful
- Suggestions of alternative measures if treatment fails

Once having chosen or been referred to a practitioner, you should have confidence in the person treating you, and you should follow any instructions given to the letter. If you receive manual therapy of any kind, you have to have faith in your practitioner in order for the treatment to work. If you are afraid or unsure during treatment, the tension generated can undermine the beneficial effects of the techniques used, even if they are perfectly chosen and performed. In order to adopt the right approach to you as an individual, your practitioner has to understand the way you feel about your problem and the treatment, so you should not be afraid to discuss any apprehensions openly. A good level of empathy between practitioner and patient is vital for the success of manual treatments.

Some patients find it easy to place complete trust in the practitioner, and therefore prefer the practitioner to maintain an element of mystery about the nature of the problem and the treatment. However, this makes it much more difficult to judge if the treatment given is appropriate. You should be given the information necessary to understand certain basic facts, so that you are in a position to make decisions about your treatment as or when appropriate. Your practitioner should be able to explain to you what could be wrong with your back or neck; what treatment methods he or she intends to use and why; what you should or may feel after a treatment session; how often treatment should be given; how many treatment sessions you are likely to need; what self-help measures you should use at each stage; what progress you can expect to make throughout the treatment programme; and what the alternatives are if the treatment fails to work.

Some factors in failed treatment

It is the practitioner's fault if:
- The assessment was inadequate
- Treatments and advice were not appropriate
- Treatments were badly performed

It is the patient's fault if:
- You fail to tell your practitioner all the relevant facts
- You fail to follow the prescribed self-help programme
- You consult several practitioners independently

Beware

Think of seeking a second opinion:
- If treatment is offered without a full physical assessment
- If your practitioner fails to answer questions adequately
- If treatment increases your symptoms or pain
- If treatment is not changed despite failing to help
- If a course of treatment is prolonged despite being unsuccessful

Important decisions have to be made if treatment fails. When treatment has not worked, you either fail to improve, or your problem gets worse. Retrogression may be a coincidence, or it may be the direct result of inappropriate treatment. There should be a safety net, if a particular line of treatment proves unable to cure your problem. Firstly, the practitioner has to be able to recognize when treatment has failed, and should not waste time and effort pursuing a line of treatment which has not improved your pain. Secondly, the practitioner should be able to suggest what needs to happen next and what you should do. It could be that you need to be referred for investigations, or to a different type of paramedic, to a medical specialist, orthopaedic surgeon or neurosurgeon. In Britain, referrals for any kind of specialist investigation and medical or surgical treatment have to be done through the general practitioner. This is one of the reasons why it is important for your paramedical practitioner to keep your doctor informed of your treatment and progress, even if you were not referred by your general practitioner in the first place.

Although treating back and neck problems is very individual when it comes to the details of treatment techniques, teamwork can be essential for correct overall care in cases where several factors are involved. When a problem is more complicated than a simple mechanical injury, different kinds of diagnostic and treatment measures may be needed. For instance, if joint disease is suspected, the general practitioner may refer the patient to a rheumatologist for investigations and treatment. In cases of severe pain, the patient may be referred to a specialist doctor or anaesthetist in case an epidural injection might help. Where appropriate, an operation may be considered, and the patient may be referred to an orthopaedic specialist or a neurosurgeon. The chronic back pain sufferer who is clinically depressed may need psychiatric treatment, perhaps with anti-depressant medication. Counselling from a clinical psychologist or psychotherapist may be needed for the depressed patient, or when excessive emotional and mental stresses affect the patient. If the patient has weight problems, food intolerances or allergies, the dietician may be able to help stabilize the situation. If poor foot function and leg length imbalance have contributed to a back problem, it may be necessary for a chiropodist or podiatrist to assess the patient and provide appropriate foot supports (orthotics) to rectify matters. Paramedics, doctors and surgeons have to co-operate when the situation demands, so there has to be good communication between the practitioners involved.

Many complementary practitioners can provide effective treatment for relieving back and neck pain, including acupuncturists, reflexologists, Shiatsu practitioners, applied kinesiologists and aromatherapists. These practitioners often work in isolation, but increasingly they are organizing themselves into teams of like-minded clinicians, frequently in conjunction with more conventionally qualified people. Many complementary techniques are now well accepted within the system of so-called conventional medicine, so that acupuncturists, for instance, may be employed in hospitals, and practitioners such as doctors and physiotherapists may learn acupuncture as an additional qualification. For postural and biomechanical correction, the Alexander technique is very widely used by all kinds of professional practitioners. The principles governing the Alexander technique were established through simple observation, but modern scientific knowledge about the central nervous system has to a large extent corroborated and justified the theories.

In most cases, the patient suffering from back or neck pain is channelled towards a physiotherapist, osteopath or chiropractor. It is not always clear to the patient or general practitioner (or indeed to the professionals themselves!) whether one of these clinicians should be chosen in preference to another in a particular situation. In combined clinics, for instance where physiotherapists work alongside osteopaths or chiropractors, it becomes easier through experiment and experience to identify which practitioner has the particular skills to help certain patients, so cross-referral between the different professionals is often practised to the benefit of the patient. Otherwise, the choice of practitioner can be a matter of guesswork, personal preference or accessibility. Individual practitioners within any profession can work to very different standards of expertise, and this is another factor to take into account. It can help to understand something about the nature of the professions and what their members are trained to do.

Physiotherapist

The scope of physiotherapy practice includes physical treatments applicable to a wide variety of problems, including chest complaints, neurological disorders, rheumatic conditions, sports injuries, and musculoskeletal problems in general. The physiotherapist's undergraduate training covers massage and manual therapy, chest physiotherapy, electrotherapy, hydrotherapy and exercise therapy. Physiotherapy patients include babies, children, adults, the old, sports stars, pregnant females, people in coma, and people with a wide variety of physical and mental disabilities.

Physiotherapy developed from a basic system of physical treatments comprising massage and exercises. The treatments were applied by prescription, under the direction of a doctor or surgeon. The British Chartered Society of Physiotherapy celebrated its centenary in 1994, and in that time the skills of the therapists have progressed together with their status. In Britain, as in many other countries in the world, chartered physiotherapists have first-contact practice, which means that they can treat patients without direct referral from a doctor. At the same time, physiotherapy has remained part of the ethical medical structure, which ensures co-operation between chartered physiotherapists and doctors and surgeons of all kinds.

The international organization of physiotherapists is the World Confederation for Physical Therapy (WCPT), which countries can join if they show that their physiotherapy training is of a high enough standard. Each country has its own governing body for physiotherapy, such as the American Physical Therapy Association (APTA), the Australian Physiotherapy Association (APA), and the Canadian Physiotherapy Association (CPA). In Britain, qualified physiotherapists are identified as members of the Chartered Society of Physiotherapy (MCSP) or as State-Registered (SRP). The national physiotherapy associations generally control training at undergraduate and postgraduate levels. They set ethical standards, and provide relevant services for their membership, such as professional indemnity insurance, legal cover and advice.

The broad base of physiotherapy training allows the practitioner to develop wide-ranging skills for treating different kinds of patient, or to specialize in techniques applicable to specific conditions. Manual therapy training for the undergraduate physiotherapist in most countries includes passive movements for the body's joints, joint mobilization techniques and a very basic grounding in manipulation. Once qualified, physiotherapists can choose to learn specialist skills. Some of the advanced skills are taught as validated postgraduate courses. In Britain, for instance, physiotherapists who have successfully completed the postgraduate manipulation course receive a diploma and are admitted to the Manipulation Association of Chartered Physiotherapists. Many MACP members join the International Federation of Orthopaedic Manipulative Therapists, through which new theories and treatment techniques from all over the world are shared and developed.

In treating back and neck problems, all qualified physiotherapists have a battery of skills which can be beneficial for the patient. Even if they have not specialized in specific advanced manipulation techniques, all trainee physiotherapists learn basic mobilization techniques for joints. Electrotherapy machines can be used variously to relieve pain and spasm and to improve function. Massage, properly applied, helps to reduce pain, decrease muscle tightness (spasm), and stimulate tissue healing processes by increasing the blood flow.

A very important element for recovery is the physiotherapist's ability to set out appropriate self-help programmes, including postural advice and remedial exercises. Physiotherapy is probably the only patient-orientated profession in which therapeutic exercise and the study of human movement (applied kinesiology) form a major part of the basic skills. Physiotherapists are therefore well placed to advise on posture, lifting techniques and correct working positions (ergonomics). They can also set out exercise programmes which can guide the patient safely from the earliest stages of a problem or immediately after an operation through to full functional recovery and a return to normal activities, whether these are intensive sports or simple recreational hobbies.

Chiropractor

Chiropractic is a profession which focuses on the relationship between impaired movement of the spinal vertebrae and the nervous system, as well as the effect such disruption may have on the patient's general health. The spinal column and pelvis have a central role in the diagnostic and therapeutic processes. The main treatment method is manipulation or 'joint adjustment', especially using short-levered high velocity thrust techniques to avoid stressing vulnerable structures unduly. Chiropractors also use other soft-tissue techniques, some electrotherapy modalities such as ultrasound and interferential therapy, rehabilitative exercises, and counselling on lifestyle factors. Drugs are not included within chiropractic treatments, although the chiropractor may refer a patient back to the general practitioner for pain-relieving medicines when appropriate.

Chiropractic is currently practised in over sixty countries worldwide, and in most places there are high standards for every chiropractor who wants a licence to practise. The first College of Chiropractic was founded as a business by a former grocer, David D. Palmer, in 1905. He had been interested in manipulative treatments for some time, and in 1895 had treated a man with neck pain following an accident some ten years previously, which had also left him deaf. Manipulative adjustment of the atlas bone not only relieved the neck pain but resulted in the patient hearing again, and so chiropractic was established.

Courses in chiropractic lasted for only two weeks at first, but were gradually extended to four years. In the United States, colleges of chiropractic are accredited through the Council of Chiropractic Education, which has been recognized by the US Department of Education since 1974. In the United States, as in Japan, the colleges are private, whereas in other countries, such as Britain, Australia, Denmark and South Africa, they have been incorporated into the university system. Graduation from the private colleges usually leads to the doctor of chiropractic degree (DC), while the graduate from the university-affiliated college is granted a bachelor of science degree in chiropractic (BSc (Chiro)).

The basic chiropractic curriculum covers all the relevant biological sciences, with special emphasis on the relationships between the musculoskeletal and nervous systems. The study of biomechanics is a major element, alongside the practical skills necessary for manual diagnosis and treatment techniques. Chiropractors are also specially trained to take and interpret X-rays as part of their diagnostic techniques. Overall, chiropractors are trained to diagnose a wide variety of complaints, and to treat many problems with manual and physical treatment techniques.

As the main treatment method applied by chiropractors is spinal manipulation, they treat any kind of derangement or dysfunction affecting the back or neck, and related problems such as referred symptoms, headaches or migraines. However, mechanical spinal problems may also be linked to other, potentially more serious conditions, although sometimes the relationship is not easy to define with certainty. Case histories illustrate the point, such as the story of the 38-year-old female patient who was treated by a chiropractor for chronic low back pain due to a degenerative L5 disc. She had also been treated for three years in in-vitro-fertilization (IVF) programmes, having been diagnosed as infertile because of 'spasm' in the smooth muscles controlling her fallopian tubes. Within a month of starting chiropractic treatment, she became pregnant. A 68-year-old male patient was treated for pain in his upper back, and found that his high blood pressure dropped from 210/140 to a respectable 150/100. Long-standing tinnitus in a 48-year-old male music teacher was greatly reduced following treatment primarily directed at the pain and tension evident in his neck and upper body. A 26-year-old female patient treated for chronic low back pain found that her irritable bowel syndrome had also improved greatly by the end of the course. Other problems which appear to benefit from chiropractic treatment include asthma and childhood bed-wetting.

Osteopath

The first serious training school for osteopaths was founded in 1897 in America by Dr Andrew Still, a general practitioner who had served as a surgeon during the American Civil War. The two-year course was gradually extended to four years, and as the profession became established Colleges of Osteopathic Medicine were gradually accepted within some American universities. In America, all osteopaths are qualified doctors, whereas in Britain osteopathy exists on two levels, as some practitioners take up the profession as qualified doctors, while others enter the profession at undergraduate level. The entry standards in both cases are high, and prospective students have to demonstrate the capacity to work effectively using their hands. In America, osteopaths have the title of Doctors of Osteopathy (DO). In Britain, osteopaths are identified as members of the London College of Osteopathic Medicine (MLCOM) and Members of the Osteopathy Register (MRO).

The traditional image of osteopaths was as 'bone-setters', but the system was always holistic and complex. The earliest osteopathic practitioners perceived the need to treat all kinds of body ailments with physical treatment techniques which would be kinder methods of promoting the body's own healing mechanisms than the more invasive, traumatic or artificial systems involved in surgery or drug-based medicine. The latter could then be reserved for the smaller number of patients who failed to respond to osteopathy techniques and who really needed surgery or drug therapy.

Because osteopathy is based on manual therapy it is logically applied to all the normal spinal problems. In technical terms, when osteopaths use high-velocity manipulation, they use what are called 'long-lever' techniques. By positioning the patient's whole body so that the target joints are very precisely placed, the osteopath can achieve a powerful unlocking motion for a particular joint without using great effort or force. Osteopathy techniques have developed and broadened over the years. Osteopaths use a huge range of techniques apart from the high-velocity manipulations which used to be considered their trade mark.

Osteopathy is applicable to a much wider range of problems than simple mechanical spinal problems. Abdominal pain is notoriously difficult for doctors to treat, as there are so many possible causes for it. The case of a 50-year-old pharmacist demonstrates how osteopathy can help. She visited her general practitioner with intense abdominal pain which had been going on for three days. The pain was vague, with no obvious signs of disease, so the GP consulted the medical osteopath in his practice. During the examination, the patient revealed that she had suffered from pain in the central area of her back (lower thoracic region) for about two weeks, but the intense abdominal pain had made her forget this, and the two pains did not seem connected. The medical osteopath treated her spine with a combination of high-velocity and gentle manipulation techniques, and used visceral manipulation directly over the abdomen. After the first session, the patient was considerably better, and she was virtually painfree following two further sessions over the next two weeks.

Sometimes conditions which can be defined but which are difficult to treat through conventional medicine can also be helped by osteopathy. One example is the case of a patient, aged 60, who suffered from Sjögren's syndrome, a rheumatological disease which gave him widespread but mild joint pains, but more disturbingly total loss of tear and saliva production. He lost all his teeth as a result, and also became very deaf in both ears. Over three years, treatment under the care of a consultant rheumatologist had failed to alleviate his symptoms, and he felt he was getting gradually worse as time went on. He used artificial tear drops to lubricate his eyes, and had to drink fluids about every ten minutes to keep his mouth moist. His condition had made him nervous, irritable and withdrawn.

In desperation, he tried many kinds of 'alternative' treatments, and eventually came under the care of a medical osteopath. The first treatment was a combination of high-velocity and gentler manipulative techniques focused on the first and second thoracic vertebrae, as they control the sympathetic nervous system, and C1 and C4 were also treated. The cranial joints close to the ear were also released. Immediately at the end of the first treatment session, he felt normal tears coming back into his eyes, and was able to stop using his eye drops from that time onwards.

Subsequent treatment sessions consisting mainly of soft-tissue techniques around the lower jaw gradually gave him a return of saliva production over the next three months. His hearing also improved, although it relapsed intermittently for no obvious reason. He attended for treatment once a fortnight, and as his condition improved his wife reported that he was much calmer, more positive and optimistic.

TREATMENTS

Traditionally, the treatment for injury pain in any part of the body was 'rest'. If a tissue caused pain, it should be protected from movement. To this end, the injured area might be immobilized. For a back injury, especially in the very painful acute stage, the whole trunk might be encased in plaster of Paris or supported in a rigid corset with metal stays. In the worst of cases, the patient might have to come to surgery, but this was very much a last resort.

More recently, practitioners have come to accept the concept that early movement following injury helps tissue healing and functional recovery. This does not mean that rest for an injured area is not used at all, but rather that movements and perhaps remedial exercises are encouraged in the patient as quickly as is safely possible. Painful activities are avoided, as pain causes inhibition, but even if the injured area itself is painful to move, it may be possible to exercise other parts of the body, to maintain general fitness and body condition, and to keep the circulation moving. In the treatment of backs and necks, techniques such as manipulation or traction which move the painful or damaged areas are now very widely used for pain relief and functional recovery.

> Dogma has no place in the treatment of back and neck problems

There are no hard-and-fast rules about which treatment method is 'right', most appropriate, or most likely to succeed for any given problem in the back or neck. The one certainty that professionals dealing with spinal problems have to share is the awareness that one cannot be dogmatic about spinal treatments. The problems are often imprecisely defined or too complex. Awareness of the technical aspects of spinal problems and the effects of treatment is increasing rapidly due to the constantly improving scientific methods for analysis. Most importantly, individual practitioners are always contributing something new to fellow practitioners.

Manual therapy

Manual therapy is the general term describing treatments in which the practitioner uses his or her hands to achieve effects on the patient's body tissues which will help to relieve the patient's problem. It includes techniques such as manipulations, mobilizations, massage, and the less conventional treatments such as Shiatsu, acupressure and reflexology. The scope of manual therapy can also be more broadly defined as including virtually all physical treatment techniques, including pain-relieving injections, but excluding surgery. All these techniques can be successful in relieving pain, reducing muscle spasm and improving joint mobility.

Practitioners learn basic manual skills by practising them under the supervision of an experienced tutor. Each practitioner then develops individual skills according to what suits his or her capabilities and personality. Many manual therapists learn techniques from practitioners in professions other than their own. Most continually update their skills by going on advanced (postgraduate or post-diploma) courses, and studying the latest articles and reference books on techniques.

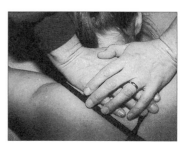

Manual therapy involves using the hands to feel and correct the patient's muscle and joint tissues

As a result, practitioners may change their methods of practice quite dramatically, sometimes several times or through many stages, during the course of their career.

Orthopaedic medicine

The late Dr James Cyriax was extremely influential in developing a system for the diagnosis and treatment of back and neck problems. He started his work, which he defined as 'orthopaedic medicine', in 1929, and his methods are still practised worldwide by doctors and physiotherapists to this day. He revolutionized the working relationships between physiotherapists and the medical profession, and encouraged physiotherapists to take up manipulation techniques, where previously their manual therapy had been largely restricted to massage and passive movements for joints.

The Society of Orthopaedic Medicine (SOM) is the existing international organization promoting and teaching treatment methods based on Dr Cyriax's principles. Its members are doctors, physiotherapists and surgeons, all of whom have equal status within the organization. The Society has close links with the British Institute of Musculoskeletal Medicine and the American Association of Orthopaedic Medicine. Joint ventures are the Journal of Orthopaedic Medicine, and the annual international conference on orthopaedic medicine.

The orthopaedic medicine treatment regime is based on a logical and very detailed assessment of the patient. In the 1975 Preface to the sixth edition of his *Textbook of Orthopaedic Medicine*, Dr Cyriax declared: 'My only important discovery, on which the whole of this work rests, is the method of systematic examination of the moving parts by selective tension'. The assessment procedures enable the practitioner to diagnose the source of a problem, especially for conditions such as intervertebral disc lesions, when X-rays usually reveal little and sophisticated scanning techniques may be inappropriate or unavailable.

The main treatment techniques used in orthopaedic medicine for back and neck problems are manipulation, traction, caudal epidural injections and sclerosing techniques. Any of these techniques can relieve the pain of a so-called 'slipped disc' or 'locked joint', and they are often used alongside other forms of therapy, such as electrotherapy, appropriate exercise programmes, advice on posture and activities, massage and medication.

In practice, manipulation will probably be the treatment of choice for the orthopaedic medicine practitioner if you have had a sudden and very acute pain, for instance when you bend down and find you are unable to straighten up again. The manipulation would consist of a short, sharp, but very small (technically tiny amplitude) movement, applied at the point where the tissue resistance is greatest. The manipulation is only applied to the part diagnosed as causing the problem, not to other parts of the spine or to the spine as a whole. The aim is to move a displaced fragment of disc, or to free a 'locked joint'. Successfully applied, the technique relieves your pain very quickly, letting you return to normal activities straight away.

If back pain and stiffness have come on the morning after a hard day's physical activity such as gardening, traction or manipulation might be the beneficial orthopaedic medicine treatment applied, after thorough examination of your spine. Traction is a mechanical stretching technique, which is usually applied daily over about two weeks in this situation.

If your back pain is agony, especially if it refers into the leg, and neither medication nor physiotherapy has helped, you might be a candidate for caudal epidural injection. This is an injection of local anaesthetic, often combined with an anti-inflammatory drug which bathes the nerve roots, reducing inflammation and pain. It is administered by a doctor who is usually a specialist in orthopaedic medicine (although other doctors outside the Society have taken up this technique), applied through a small opening at the very base of your tailbone (coccyx). Surgery is usually considered when back pain is extreme, but a successful caudal epidural injection may avoid the need for an operation. The injection can also work well for long-term (chronic) back pain, or for sciatica, which may be causing leg numbness or weakness.

Sometimes, a back problem keeps recurring, even though medication and physiotherapy relieve it apparently successfully at each episode. This problem is defined as an 'unstable back', which may well be helped by sclerosing therapy. This is a course of usually three injections of a 'sugar' solution into the ligaments which support the low back. The effect is to tighten the ligaments so that they act as an 'internal corset' which prevents any structures from moving out of place and causing problems.

Manipulation

Manipulation simply means 'to work with the hands', or 'to handle', and this vague overall meaning has left the term open to a wide interpretation when it is used to specify a therapeutic technique. In the broadest sense, it can mean any passive movement performed by a practitioner to create an increase of joint movement or tissue mobility in the patient. In the context of spinal problems, manipulation can be defined as a rapid (high-velocity) thrust performed by the practitioner to create a very small movement at the end of a joint's available range. This distinguishes manipulation from mobilization, which is a much milder technique performed at low velocity using any part of a joint's range.

Advances in manipulative treatment methods have been due to the specialist practitioners who have passed on their individual expertise in treating patients through clinical teaching textbooks and manuals for the guidance of current and future practitioners. Doctors, surgeons, physiotherapists, osteopaths, chiropractors and other practitioners have contributed to the development of treatment methods for spinal problems beyond simple immobilization or complicated surgery. Their names are familiar outside their own professions to most practitioners specializing in the treatment of back and neck injuries. Among the best known, past and present, are Professor J. Bourdillon, Mr David Butler, Dr James Cyriax, Dr Viola Frymann, Mr Gregory Grieve, Dr Vladimir Janda, Dr Freddy Kaltenborn, Dr Karel Lewit, Mr Geoffrey Maitland, Mr Brian Mackenzie, Dr James Mennell, Mr Brian Mulligan, Dr Christine O'Donoghue, Dr Andrew Still and Dr Alan Stoddard, but there are many others around the world.

Full-thrust manipulation, if applied successfully, creates an immediate improvement of joint movement and freedom, which is obviously beneficial in cases where joint stiffness or 'locking' have been a problem. Manipulative techniques can be directed precisely to single joints, or performed in such a way as to move several joints more or less at once. The exact effects of manipulation are not known in detail, but it can release minor adhesions (tissues which have become tight or 'stuck'), relieve muscle spasm, and move a loose body within a joint. The idea that manipulation works by putting structures such as discs 'back into place' is slightly misleading. Manipulation which releases tight structures can create better bone and joint alignment, and its main effect is to increase your overall range of movement.

Because of its dramatic effects, manipulation is often perceived as an instant 'magic cure' by patients and practitioners alike. More dangerously, unqualified people sometimes learn a few techniques and use them without any awareness of the many possible reasons for *not* manipulating a spine in certain situations. I have known of sports coaches 'treating' their athletes with full-thrust manipulations. This is simply irresponsible.

Even when used by qualified practitioners, there are some risks attached to full-thrust manipulation. If it is applied in the wrong situation, for instance if there is malignant disease in the spine, it can cause damage. It is also vital for manipulation to be applied against a background of protective exercises. An appropriate level of joint stability has to be achieved through remedial exercises and bad postural habits must be corrected. If not, the overall result of a course of manipulation can be progressive joint instability, which is usually coupled with increasing pain, even if treatment sessions seem to provide immediate relief at the time. It is especially likely to happen if manipulation is repeated too frequently. Painful instability can also result from manipulation of healthy symptom-free joints. Personally, I believe that manipulation of healthy joints is neither effective nor appropriate as a measure for preventing spinal problems.

Manipulation under anaesthetic (MUA) is a technique used mainly by orthopaedic surgeons to free joints which have been stiff and painful for a long time, or which have become fixed in position. With the patient unconscious, there is no muscular resistance to the forced movement, so a good joint range can be achieved. MUA is not used very much for spinal joints. The advantage of normal manipulation is that the tissue response to every technique applied can be assessed for their good or bad effects immediately, and the patient remains in ultimate control of the treatment, except at the instant when the manipulation is applied.

Mobilizations and related manipulative techniques

Mobilization techniques are gentle forms of manipulation performed as rocking (oscillating) movements within a joint's painless range. Mobilizations are always very precisely directed to a specific joint, and they can achieve pain relief, improvement in the blood circulation, improvement in the fluid balance within the intervertebral discs, and reduction of any muscle spasm around the joint. The techniques are not as dramatic in effect as full-thrust manipulations, but they can be as beneficial. Many patients find the gentler form of treatment less frightening and more reassuring, as they can feel that they are in control of the situation throughout the whole treatment.

There are many developments in physical treatments which have grown out of existing theories and methods of practice. The use of combined movements as a system for assessing spinal problems has been a refinement of standard movement testing procedures, due to the observation that normally movements in the spine do not occur only in one plane, but as combinations across planes. By identifying which combinations of movements reproduce the patient's symptoms, the practitioner can choose appropriate treatment techniques for manipulating the joints so that they regain the necessary freedom to move without causing pain.

Unlike forms of manipulation based on quick or slow movements in a joint, SNAGs (sustained natural apophyseal glides) are mobilizing techniques which are carried out at the limit of the movement range with sustained pressure on the joint being treated. A completely unique feature of the system is the fact that all the mobilizations are performed with the joint in a weight-bearing position, so the patient is sitting or standing up, whereas for most other forms of manual therapy the patient usually lies down, and only rarely sits or stands during the treatment. The patient may co-operate with the mobilization techniques by performing appropriate active movements according to instruction. SNAGs can also be self-applied as a home-treatment technique by the patient, once the practitioner has shown the patient exactly what to do.

'Functional techniques' are another version of manual therapy which use slow, sustained movements in a very small range to promote relaxation and freedom in a stiff, painful spinal joint. Linked to these are 'muscle energy techniques' in which the patient actively contracts the muscles controlling a painful joint against the movement which the therapist initiates. This is similar to the principles of proprioceptive neuro-muscular facilitation (PNF) (see p.202) and can be very effective in restoring joint movement without creating instability. Modifications of muscle energy techniques can improve stability when a joint is abnormally lax.

Traditionally, manipulation and mobilization techniques aimed to move joints in order to affect their mechanical systems. More recently, treatment techniques have been directed towards the nervous system itself, as practitioners have become aware that the body's nerve systems can also suffer from functional disturbance when the spinal joints have been damaged. Special tests and treatment techniques for the nervous system have been developed within a treatment regime usually referred to as 'adverse neural tension' (ANT).

Craniosacral therapy is a treatment concept developed over more than fifty years. It started as part of osteopathy, but is now increasingly used by many other manual therapists from different disciplines. It is based on the principle that the meningeal membranes and the cerebrospinal fluid in the central nervous system, together with all the structures closely related to them, constitute the craniosacral system. This system exerts an influence on all the major body systems, which is reciprocated. It has its own inherent rhythm, a pulsation which is normally between six and twelve cycles per minute. Craniosacral therapists use this rhythm in applying gentle non-invasive manipulative techniques with the aim of restoring normal physiological movement to an area which is disturbed or inhibited in some way.

Traction

The simple definition of traction in the therapeutic context is pulling joints slightly apart. The aim of traction is to relieve pressure on joint structures, to improve fluid flow through the joints, and to reduce tension in the spinal muscles. It can help relieve pain, and can be particularly effective in relieving the referred symptoms which indicate that nerve function has been disrupted.

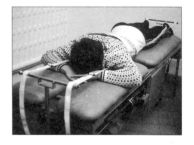

Lumbar traction. The spinal stretch is done with the patient lying face down or face up, according to the condition

There are many different ways of applying traction. It can be applied manually by the practitioner, so that it is in fact a manipulative technique. It can also be applied mechanically, using a harness or head halter and straps and a system to exert leverage on the spinal joints. The system may work as a simple pulley attached to weights, or it may use an electric motor which delivers a certain level of tension through the cords attached to the harness or head halter. The amount of tension generated is usually calculated in pounds or kilogrammes, and is determined by the practitioner.

For very acute back or neck pain, especially in cases where there is also referred pain into the arm(s) or leg(s), the patient is sometimes admitted to hospital and put on continuous traction for a few days or sometimes even weeks. Although the patient is allowed to get up to wash and go to the toilet, he or she is expected to remain lying down for most of the day. More usually, traction is applied using a special treatment couch designed so that the patient can be placed in a comfortable position and the stretch can be achieved at the appropriate level of the spine. On a traction couch the stretch can be given as intermittent or constant. Intermittent traction has timed stretching and relaxation phases, which may be set at perhaps 30 seconds or one minute each. When the traction is constant, the stretch is held for a set period, perhaps 20 or 30 minutes. The poundage may be very light at first, so that not much seems to happen, and then it is gradually increased, either within the treatment session or on successive treatments. Mechanical traction may be repeated on a daily basis, or less frequently, perhaps once or twice a week, according to the practitioner's judgement.

Injection

Any injection is an invasive procedure, in that the needle has to be inserted accurately into the body, so that it reaches the part where it is supposed to do good, and avoids other parts, which may be very close to the target tissue, where it might cause damage.

Apart from accuracy of delivery, the person administering the injection has to be aware of the substance being injected, what dosage is needed in a given situation, what effect the substance can have on the tissues, any side-effects it could have, and what alternatives could be used if the patient is allergic to it. In most countries, pain-relieving or anti-inflammatory injections are supposed to be administered only by medically qualified people (doctors and surgeons). In some countries, suitably qualified and experienced paramedics such as physiotherapists are legally and ethically entitled to give injections under a doctor's supervision.

In practice, in many countries, it is not uncommon for paramedics to use injections as part of their range of treatments. Some paramedical professions define this as being within their stated scope of practice, whereas in others the use of injections by members of the professional association has caused debate about whether the profession should widen its remit to include such procedures. Ethically, if a practitioner performs a procedure outside the scope of his or her professional practice, it is not covered under professional liability insurance. If anything goes wrong, this can be highly damaging to the patient's interests.

From the patient's point of view, the most important issues are whether an injection is administered under the safest possible conditions; whether it is appropriate for the problem and likely to be of benefit; and whether the person administering the injection is qualified, experienced and expert enough to do it efficiently.

Surgery

Surgery is the last resort, when conservative treatment has failed. For severe back pain, especially associated with sciatica, which nothing seems to relieve, the cause of the nerve compression is identified, usually through an MRI scan. The patient may then be considered for surgery, and assessed by an orthopaedic specialist or neurosurgeon. The surgeon will consider it vital to select the patient with care, to avoid unnecessary or unhelpful procedures.

If the spine is unstable, it may be made secure with corrective surgery, but this is very rare. Chemonucleolysis is a surgical technique in which the enzyme chymopapain is administered to try to dissolve parts of an intervertebral disc, to reduce the pressure it can exert against the nerve root. This technique is used more frequently in America than in Britain, as is laser discotomy, a relatively new technique in which the surgeon uses a laser or cutting blade to remove the damaged area of the disc from the inside in an attempt to reduce the pressure inside the disc and make the prolapse retract.

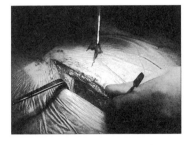

Open discectomy: removal of a damaged disk by cutting into the back through a scar (incision)

If the nerve is being compressed by a degenerate or damaged disc, the most widely used operation to solve the problem is the discectomy, or disc removal. The modern technique is to do this through an operating microscope (microdiscectomy), so that there is only a tiny scar (incision) and as little disruption to the area as possible.

If the cause of the nerve compression proves to be spinal stenosis (see p.141), the narrow spinal canal is widened through an operation called a laminectomy.

The patient is usually up and about within a few days of surgery, or as quickly as pain and the general recovery from the anaesthetic permit. A progressive rehabilitation programme is usually recommended to help the patient recover full function.

Electrotherapy

Electrotherapy is the use of machines for various beneficial effects, including pain relief, tissue healing, reduction of fluid swelling in joints, improvement of muscle function together with neuromuscular co-ordination. Some electrotherapy modalities work passively, like ultrasound and laser therapy, which can help to relieve pain and swelling, and to speed up healing of damaged tissue to a slight extent. These machines have to be used very precisely. The therapist has to choose the appropriate dosage and use it at the right stage of the injury only on those tissues which are known to benefit. It is also important to know when not to use these modalities. For instance, ultrasound is thought to be possibly harmful to growing bone ends (epiphyses) in the young, and it is *never* used if there is the slightest possibility that the patient might have malignant disease.

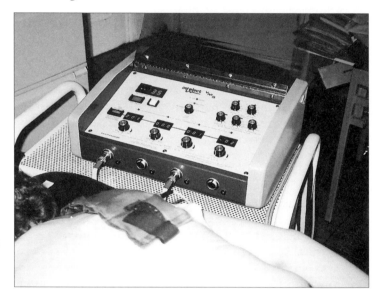

Electrical muscle stimulation for the upper back muscles. The electrodes are held in place by a light weight, which also acts as a resistance when the patient lifts the upper back as the electrical current activates the muscles

Electrical currents, including those produced in Interferential and Diadynamic therapy can be used to relieve pain, improve circulatory flow, reduce muscle tightness and improve muscle function. TENs (transcutaneous electrical nerve stimulation) is one of the most widely used electrical pain-relieving modalities. It may be used as treatment by the practitioner, and the patient may also be taught how to use one of these tiny machines for self-help pain relief over several hours each day.

Biofeedback provides information about the level of activity in a muscle. It uses a low-frequency electrical current which picks up the muscle's degree of tension and transmits an audible signal. The more tense the muscle, the louder the signal. Biofeedback is used to help the patient become aware of muscle tightness or flabbiness (low tone), in order to adjust by relaxing or activating the muscle according to the signal provided by the biofeedback machine. Like TENs, biofeedback can be used for professional treatment or as a self-help technique.

Electrical muscle stimulation can be used to improve neuromuscular co-ordination, reduce muscle spasm and help muscle function. As pain and injuries inevitably cause inhibition in nerve-muscle function, I use electrical muscle stimulation routinely to restore precise muscle action following a physical problem, especially in the muscles of the back.

Exercise therapy

All treatments for back and neck problems aim to remove the obstacles which prevent functional movement and activity. These may be pain; poor nerve function; tight, weak or inhibited muscles; or stiff or 'locked' joints. Once they have been removed, bad habits in posture and movement have to be eradicated, and normal patterns restored. There are situations in which exercise is contra-indicated, most notably if there is a major disc prolapse with severe nerve disruption (neurological signs). In all cases, if exercises seem to be making a problem worse, they have to be modified or discontinued until the situation changes, making exercise safe for the patient.

Remedial exercises are vital for recovering good quality of movement for normal physical function. All remedial exercises are set with the specific aims of maintaining and improving muscle strength and flexibility, increasing joint mobility and stability, regaining co-ordinated action between the injured area and surrounding parts, and making normal physical activities possible again. The exercises are tailored to the individual, the condition, the stage of the problem, the rate of recovery, and the degree of recovery.

When remedial exercises are appropriate, they are always precise and progressive. They should never cause pain during or after a session, nor should they be too demanding for the patient to perform easily and comfortably. Remedial exercises should almost feel too easy, as though they were not achieving anything. Active sports players sometimes find this difficult to understand, as they are used to feeling immediate effects from exercise. However, remedial exercises should never involve effort or forceful movements.

Different practitioners use various exercise regimes for spinal problems. There are many different types of exercise which can be done for the spine, from many different starting positions. A selection is given in chapter 9. My own programmes use stabilizing exercises as the basis for activity. These are usually very small-range movements, partly to achieve the maximum stabilizing effect, and partly to avoid causing pain in any of the joints. Performing the movements slowly against gravity is an important element in improving postural muscle tone and joint stability. Once a good level of stability has been gained and the pain threshold is receding, I add exercises designed to improve overall spinal mobility. In order to avoid the risk of destabilizing any vulnerable joints, I usually set exercises which combine mobility with co-ordination. In the final stages of rehabilitation for sports players, the remedial exercises may become more demanding in order to blend into normal training routines.

For all patients following an active rehabilitation programme, a basic schedule of simple remedial exercises is maintained throughout the whole recovery period. Patients are encouraged to keep up the discipline indefinitely, if possible, so that the basic remedial exercises serve in the long term as protective exercises for preventing further problems.

An appropriate exercise programme, like any other treatment modality, may have to be devised according to careful analysis of the problem. In one instance, a 42-year-old patient had had a very difficult pregnancy. The baby had lain sideways inside the womb, and the obstetrician had tried pummelling the mother's abdomen in an unsuccessful attempt to turn him. He was then born by Caesarean section and weighed in at 9 lbs. Following this, the mother's abdomen had remained extremely tender. She could not lie face down, even the slightest pressure hurt, and coughing and sneezing were especially painful.

Two years after the birth, there was a noticeable 4-inch (approximately 10-centimetre) 'gap' between her abdominal muscles on each side. The muscles were very flabby, protruding and extremely weak. The mother felt her back was increasingly vulnerable, and it had started to 'go' when she picked her son up. She had been given abdominal strengthening exercises to do, but despite trying hard she found them difficult to achieve, and her abdominal tenderness had only eased slightly during that time. The patient was referred to me by her general practitioner. On assessment, I found that she had a generalized loss of co-ordination and balance, and some differences in her ability to perform movements with her right and left leg. Therefore, I set out an exercise programme of co-ordinated exercises, some of which would activate the abdominal muscles indirectly. The basic exercises set were: standing, going up and down on the toes; balancing on one leg; balancing on one leg and hip hitching (see p.196); stomach-lying trunk and hip extension; and half-crook-lying hip extension (see p.162).

Three weeks later, the patient was feeling better and the tenderness in her abdomen had eased significantly. Her abdominal muscles had gained some tone, they looked flatter, and she was able to contract them. I did one session of electrical muscle stimulation with active movements directly for the abdominal muscles.

One month after this, having continued the exercise programme including direct abdominal strengthening exercises (see pp.156–60), the patient was very much better, and the 'gap' between the abdominal muscles was smaller. At this stage, she was no longer having any episodes of back pain. She was set a final-stage programme to pursue over the next few months, consisting of the basic programme of exercises, a new exercise for her oblique abdominal muscles, and regular use of a muscle stimulator combined with active movements to continue the improvement in her abdominal muscles.

As she had been told by several practitioners that they could do nothing to help her problems of pain and weakness, this patient was delighted to find that a comprehensive 'self-help' programme of appropriate exercises could bring her back to normal.

THE TREATMENT PROGRAMME

Treatment for spinal problems is almost always a combination of different techniques and types of therapy. Pain-relieving electrotherapy modalities may be given in the same treatment session as manual therapy techniques. Different treatments may be used in successive sessions, or the practitioner may construct a pattern of treatment which is maintained throughout the whole course. Changes in treatment modalities depend on how you respond to each type of treatment, on the outcome of each treatment session, and on how well you get on with any self-help regime you have been advised to do in between sessions.

How often treatment is given to a particular patient

depends on the practitioner's preference, what the problem is, and what stage it is at. For the patient who has been admitted to hospital with an acute problem, pain-relieving physical treatments may be given several times every day, or treatment may be restricted to drugs and bed-rest. In the acute phase of a problem which is treated in a hospital out-patients' department, clinic or practice, treatment may be given on a daily basis, or spread out on the basis of one or more sessions per week. There may be good reasons for intensive daily treatments in the later stages of a problem. If you have chronic back pain, for instance, and you have received a lot of treatment over a long time, your practitioner may decide to give you a full daily programme of treatment over a short period such as a fortnight or one month. This is usually done within the framework of a Pain Clinic, with several practitioners involved, and you are likely to be admitted as an in-patient for the course, although it can also be done on an out-patient basis.

Essential elements of rehabilitation treatment for full functional recovery

- An appropriate remedial exercise programme
- Posture correction

In most cases, if at all possible, I prefer to spread out treatment sessions for my back and neck patients, seeing them about once a week at first, and then perhaps fortnightly or monthly. In the sessions, I use some electrotherapy modalities, sometimes traction, but mainly manual therapy techniques. My preference is for the gentlest type of manual therapy, to give the patient confidence in the healing and recovery processes. Patients rarely respond positively to treatments which scare them. In the case of children and young patients, treatment should probably always be carefully conservative, as we do not know the exact effects of many forms of electrotherapy or of techniques such as full-thrust manipulations on growing bones and joints. In virtually every case, I try to give all my patients a comprehensive programme of self-help mea-

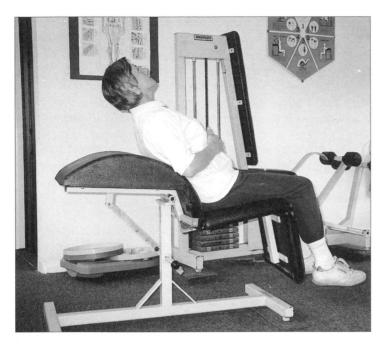

The Norsk abdominal exerciser: the abdominal muscles are put on the stretch and strengthened, keeping the back arched. The hips are bent to prevent too much activity in the hip flexor muscles

sures, postural advice and progressive remedial exercises, in order to achieve the best possible level of functional recovery.

The patient has to be responsible for carrying out the instructions given, as in the long term it is up to the patient to learn to look after his or her spine and protect it from further problems where possible. In the case of young patients, the parent or guardian has to ensure that the programme is followed accurately. Spacing out the treatment sessions allows time for the remedial exercise programme to have its

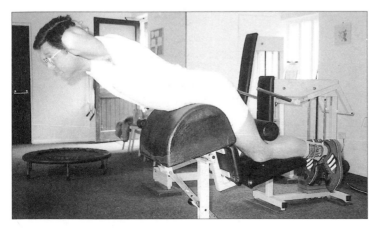

The Norsk back extension machine, designed to work the back extensor muscles through a safe range of movement using gravity as the resistance

effect. The patient's progress can be monitored over several weeks so that setbacks can be analysed and corrected, and good exercise and postural habits instilled and reinforced.

During the recovery phase, I usually encourage the patient to use an exercise gymnasium, preferably using the Norsk Sequence-Training rehabilitation machines. The controlled workout is suitable for all types of patient, from serious athletes to people who have never done formal exercise training before. Physical training gives the patient a sense of well-being, and is vital for achieving peak physical condition. Properly tailored, it is appropriate for all age groups and all types of patient, from the very young to the elderly.

Spinal conditions and diagnosis

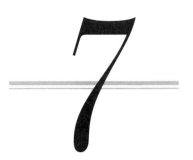

DIAGNOSIS

A great many things can go wrong with the back and neck. Knowing how an injury has happened does not necessarily establish what type of damage has been sustained. There are many structures in the back and neck which can be broken, torn or strained, and it is not always clear whether one or many tissues might be involved through any particular injury. If the injury cause is not known, the situation is even worse. Unfortunately, pain patterns do not identify what is wrong. Pain may even be misleading. A lot of pain does not necessarily mean a major problem; conversely, little pain does not guarantee that the problem is only minor. The place where you feel the pain is not necessarily the source, nor does it identify which parts or structures in the back or neck are involved.

It is very important to understand that diagnosis of back and neck problems is a complex and specialized task. The first priority is to identify whether your problem is a mechanical injury or due to other causes, such as disease. In many, if not most cases of mechanical injury, the practitioner may not know precisely what is causing the pain or symptoms. It is impossible to be certain which structures are involved or how badly they are damaged without specialist investigations. However, being certain of the precise nature of the damage is not always essential to successful treatment. Treatment is very often, quite reasonably, based on probability. In most cases investigations are not needed, and problems can be solved by treatment based on the clinical signs and symptoms which the practitioner has observed through examining you.

Among the many investigations which can be done, most have disadvantages as well as advantages, so they will only be ordered by the doctor in charge of your case if they are considered absolutely essential.

X-rays simply show up the bones, so they reveal any abnormalities in the formation or position of the spinal bones. Generally, X-rays are less used now than previously, partly because the information they give is limited, and partly to avoid any possible risks associated with over-exposing the patient to potentially harmful radiation. A more precise, but invasive investigation is the myelogram, for which a special type of dye (contrast medium) is injected into the spinal canal, in order to help identify problems such as a prolapsed disc or spinal stenosis. One of the major drawbacks of the myelogram has been that it can cause very severe headaches afterwards, according to the type of contrast medium used.

More modern diagnostic techniques, such as Computerized Axial Tomography (CAT or CT scans) and Magnetic Resonance Imaging (MRI), can provide an accurate picture of damaged tissues in many cases. However, such tests are expensive.

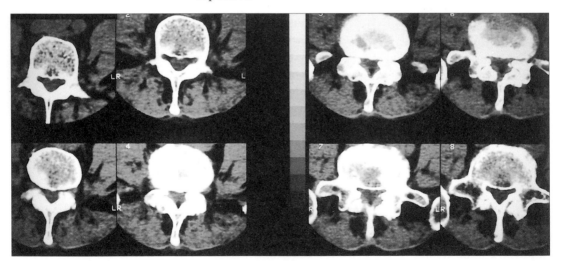

CT scan showing spinal stenosis in the lumbar canal (see p.141)

Other investigations may be used with or without specific investigations for the spine itself. In many cases, your doctor may order blood tests to find out whether you could have inflammation, infection or perhaps disease in your system. If you have referred symptoms into an arm or leg which indicate nerve root disruption, you may be referred for nerve conduction tests. These are electrical measurements showing how efficiently your nerves are activating your muscles in each part of the affected area.

Diagnosis is certainly not something you can do for yourself, however well you think you know your own body, or however much you might be persuaded that because your pain is identical to another patient's, it must be the same injury in need of the same treatment.

I vividly remember the case of an athlete, J., whom I had treated intermittently for occasional injuries over a space of about two years. He competed in throwing events, and had previously fractured his backbone in a parachuting accident, which had partially paralysed him at the time, but from which he had fully recovered. One evening he came into my clinic after a heavy training session. He was bent over in acute pain, apparently from his lower back. He begged me to manipulate his back, saying that his osteopath always put him right in this way whenever he had an acute back spasm. Rather than manipulate, I recommended that J. get himself taken home, apply ice to the painful area, rest, and call his doctor if the pain persisted. He did as I suggested, and was sent to hospital when his pain failed to subside. An X-ray revealed that he had fractured the top of his thigh-bone (femur). It was not clear how the injury had happened, although it was possible that J. had suffered a stress fracture in the neck of the femur through overtraining, and this had fractured completely that evening under the strain of further training repetitions. Fortunately, the bone healed perfectly, and after a few months J. was able to resume his sports without further problems.

THE ASSESSMENT PROCESS

Identifying the source of the pain is crucial to solving any problem, which will not be solved just by treating the mechanical symptoms. The main method of identifying what is wrong is through the clinical history, or your description of what has happened. The process of unravelling cause and effect in any kind of spinal problem is simpler and quicker if you describe your problem lucidly - and very slow if you don't. You have to be prepared to state all the necessary facts, preferably in chronological order. Your practitioner has to take an accurate history of what has happened to you, what you have felt, and all your symptoms, even if they seem to you totally unconnected to your spinal pain. Both practitioner and patient have to be prepared to go through a detailed process of questions and answers, if the pain pattern does not at first add up logically to a reasonable conclusion of what might be wrong. In the majority of cases, the clinical history is the basis for the physical examination and treatment, although in a few cases it can indicate that diagnostic investigations are required.

Questions the practitioner may ask you

In taking your general details, the practitioner usually establishes exactly how old you are, and what you do routinely each day, whether you are a student, housewife, office worker, manual worker or professional sports player. You will probably be asked to describe the movements or postures your daily activities involve. The practitioner also needs to know what your leisure activities are, whether these are sedentary or involve active sports. If you do one or more sports, go to exercise classes, or use exercise video tapes, you will be asked how often you participate.

The questions asked will depend on the practitioner, and to a certain extent on the patient. If the patient is a very young child, the questioning will be kept to a minimum, and it is up to the parent or responsible adult to be prepared to answer necessary background questions if possible. For the older child or teenager, it is often best to let them speak for themselves if they have to attend for treatment. Even if the young patient is shy at first, it helps to establish confidence in the practitioner if the child is allowed to describe the problem in his or her own terms. The immediate communication also makes the child more aware of what is happening and more 'in charge' of the situation, so that attending for physical treatment may perhaps seem less daunting than visiting a hospital clinic or a dental surgery.

The adult patient should prepare as well as possible for the assessment. If you have kept an accurate diary of your symptoms, you can show it to the practitioner, or even send a brief account of the problem in advance, if there is sufficient time before you attend for your appointment. The practitioner will then have background knowledge on which to base further inquiries. Of the questions which may be asked, some will be elaborated if the answers lead to other questions or possibilities, whereas others may be omitted if they become irrelevant in the light of the information given. In general, you can expect to be asked at least some of the following questions.

1. What is the problem?
- Do you have pain in your back or neck?
- If so, is it in the middle, to one side, or right across?
- Do you have pain, tingling or numbness in your arm(s) or leg(s)?
- If you have referred symptoms, do they seem connected to your neck or back?

2. What is the history of the problem?
- When did it start?
- Did it start suddenly, for a known reason?
- Did it come on gradually?
- What were you doing when it started?
- Was there any change in your routine which could have caused the problem?
- Have you had the same problem before?
- Have you had different symptoms affecting the same region before?

3. What is the daily pain pattern?
- Do you have pain all the time?
- Do you have pain on certain movements or activities?
- Do you wake up during the night in pain?
- Does your spine feel especially stiff or painful in the morning?
- Do your symptoms ease during the day?
- Do your symptoms feel worse in the evening?

4. Is your pain related to your activities or posture?
- Do you feel pain or other symptoms sitting down, standing up, driving or walking?
- Do you feel pain or other symptoms at rest?
- Do you feel increased pain during or after physical activities?
- Can you lie comfortably a) on your back, b) on your stomach or c) on your side?
- Do you have pain when you cough or sneeze?

5. Is your general health good?
- Have you ever had any major or significant illnesses?
- Have you had any illnesses or infections recently?

- Were you ill around the time your problem started?
- Have you been feeling run-down or especially tired?
- Have you had any problems passing urine or bowel motions?
- Have you had constipation or diarrhoea?
- Do you suffer from any allergies or known food intolerances?
- Is there any family history of arthritic or other illnesses?
- (Females) Have you had any kind of hormonal problems or changes?
- Are you taking any kinds of medicine for any reason?

6. What is your lifestyle like?
- Do you work long hours?
- Do you travel a lot?
- If you do sport seriously, how much do you do?
- Do you take regular general exercise?
- Do you allow time to rest and relax every day?
- What do you do for relaxation or recreation?
- Do you eat regular meals, including varied foods and fresh vegetables?
- Do you drink plenty of plain water every day?
- How much tea or coffee do you drink, if any?
- Do you drink alcohol: never, rarely, regularly, in moderation, or in excess?
- Have you been under particular pressures at work or at home?
- Have you suffered any bereavements or other emotional upsets?

THE PHYSICAL EXAMINATION

When the practitioner has gained the necessary background knowledge about the nature and extent of your current problem, and any underlying factors which might influence it, you will be physically examined. For this, the practitioner usually asks you to undress down to your underwear. You should be prepared for this, and wear suitable garments. If preferred, men can wear swimming trunks and women a bikini. A one-piece swimsuit or all-in-one 'body' is not suitable for the physical examination or treatment. If you are embarrassed by the prospect of taking your outer clothes off, perhaps if you have a skin complaint on your chest or back, you should explain this to your practitioner. You may be able to keep a vest on during the examination, although your practitioner may need to lift it a little in order to be able to see or feel specific parts of your back or neck. If your practitioner works alone, but you would prefer a second person to be present while you are undressed, you should make this clear. If someone has come with you to your appointment, perhaps a spouse, relative or friend, you should also make it clear before the start whether you prefer the person to be present or not during the assessment and examination.

There are many different tests for assessing spinal problems, and they are chosen according to the situation. Many practitioners have their own individual ways of testing joints, and their preferred order of performing physical tests. In general, the tests most practitioners use aim to assess your active joint movements, muscle balance, muscle strength, passive joint movements, how tender and sensitive your joint structures are, how your joint tissues and muscles feel to the touch, whether your reflexes are working normally, whether your nervous system is functioning efficiently, and whether your skin sensation is normal. With each test your practitioner assesses what the reaction is by watching, touching or both, and you should say if you feel particular pain at any time. You may be unable to perform some of the movements required because of pain or restriction. All your reactions are noted down for future reference.

There are innumerable tests for the biomechanical systems, including the exercise tests listed in chapter 8 (see pp. 156–78). The practitioner will choose those which are most relevant to the symptoms you have described.

Some tests are done standing up, usually with the practitioner watching how your joints move while guiding the movements at the same time. The practitioner may press you in the direction of the movement when you have reached your normal limit. This is called adding over-pressure. You may be asked to bend backwards, forwards and sideways to check the movements of your spine as a whole and especially your low back. After the basic movements which happen more or less in straight lines, you may have to do combined movements such as twisting and bending.

Sitting upright on the side of the treatment couch is another position in which biomechanical movements can be checked. The twisting movements of your upper back, and all the movements of your neck can be tested in this position.

The practitioner may also guide you to extend and bend your spine straightening up and relaxing, or into a sideways movement from the pelvis upwards.

Palpation is the technical term for assessing the tissues through feeling them. The practitioner usually palpates the back and neck as you go through the movement tests standing and sitting. When you are lying down on your stomach, the practitioner can feel your spinal muscles and assess whether they are in spasm (over-tense) or flabby (low-tone). With precise manipulation of the spinal joints, the practitioner can feel correct or inefficient joint movement, blockage in any part of the normal movement range, tenderness in any of the bones when they are touched, or a painful reaction to normal pressure against a joint on a particular movement. When you lie on your back, the practitioner can check your hip and shoulder mobility, to assess whether there is any abnormality of movement, or whether your symptoms can be reproduced from these joints.

Testing various aspects of the nervous system is an important element in the physical assessment. Your reflexes may be tested by tapping your tendons lightly with a special rubber hammer, especially at your knees, ankles, elbows and wrists.

Skin sensation may be tested anywhere over your back, neck, legs or arms by touching different areas lightly with sharp and blunt objects alternately to see if you can detect the difference with your eyes closed. Some co-ordination tests may also be done with your eyes closed, such as touching your thumbs to each finger on the same hand in turn, or touching different parts of your head or body with your hand on command.

There are many different manoeuvres to stretch the nerves in order to show whether they are working efficiently or not. Traditional tests include the straight-leg-raise and the femoral nerve stretch test. For the straight-leg-raise test you lie on your back and the practitioner lifts one of your legs upwards with the knee straight. If there is painful restriction down the back of the leg on one side, it may be due to nerve root compression. Sometimes the pain is relieved if the practitioner pulls gently on your leg, applying traction away from your trunk. The pain may be increased if you are asked to lift your head forwards, or if the practitioner presses against your foot to bring your toes towards your body (into ankle dorsiflexion). Sometimes the straight-leg-raise causes pain in your back, with or without accompanying leg pain. The back pain may be on the same or the opposite side as the leg being lifted.

The femoral nerve stretch test is done as you lie on your stomach. The practitioner gently bends each knee individually to its limit, and then both knees simultaneously. You may feel pain along the front of one thigh relative to the other, back pain on the same or opposite side when one leg is under test, or back pain centrally or to one side when both knees are bent together.

Tension tests for the nervous system have been developed and refined in relation to the Adverse Neural Tension (ANT) system of treatment. Passive Neck Flexion is a test usually performed while you lie on your back. You raise your head a little, and the practitioner then gently bends your neck a little further passively. This test can identify problems with the nerves not only in the neck, but also lower down the spine. The Slump Test is performed with you sitting on the side of the couch with your hands behind your back. There are various stages, starting with bending your back and your neck. You then straighten your knee and foot one at a time at first, then both legs together. At each stage the practitioner adds slight over-pressure, and carefully assesses any response of pain or change in your symptoms.

A series of tests has been developed for the various nerves which come out of the neck region into the arm, and these are called Upper Limb Tension Tests (ULTTs). Most are done with the patient lying supine (on the back), although a different position, such as stomach-lying, may be chosen for a specific reason. The tests consist of placing one arm in a stretched position, either sideways, upwards or downwards away from your body, and then increasing the tension by applying some extra pressure to the shoulder, elbow or hand. Further tension can be exerted through the nervous system if an assistant practitioner helps you to add the straight-leg-raise movement while the stretched position of the arm is maintained.

PROBLEMS IN THE BACK AND NECK

Countless problems can affect the spinal joints. It is important to understand this, so that you do not draw hasty conclusions and try to diagnose your own problem. Spinal problems can be divided into mechanical problems, inflammatory and metabolic diseases, and infections, illnesses and viruses, which can all separately cause apparently similar symptoms affecting the back or neck.

As in other parts of the body, an injury or painful condition can arise from bones, muscles, ligaments, discs, joint capsules, nerves, in fact any of the structural tissues. In the spine, however, it is rare for one tissue alone to be the sole cause of pain. If a bone or one of the joint structures is damaged or painful, for instance, the muscles overlying the joint are likely to go into spasm and add to the pain. If a spinal muscle is strained or torn, the joint(s) which it controls may be blocked, possibly causing secondary strain of the joint structures.

Some of the conditions which occur within each category are listed below, in alphabetical order, so that you understand what can happen and what to expect if you have been told that you suffer from one of these problems. Do not make the mistake of reading through the list and identifying your own symptoms with each and every problem. Mistaken self-diagnosis can really get you down, which does not help you to help yourself. Leave diagnosis and treatment to those with professional expertise, preferably a team of practitioners whom you can trust.

MECHANICAL PROBLEMS

Any of the spinal tissues can be damaged through traumatic or overuse injury, causing pain and functional disturbance. The terms used to describe mechanical problems can be vague, which reflects the fact that the precise nature of the damage often remains unknown.

Disc problems

When an intervertebral disc has become damaged or broken it is technically described as *prolapsed* or *herniated*. These terms are usually applied in the situation when the nucleus pulposus has broken through the containing structure provided by the annulus fibrosus. Once there is a major disruption, other material besides the nucleus pulposus can be involved, such as fibres from the annulus, or parts of the cartilage end-plate from the vertebral body. If the herniation is central, and the nucleus is pushed backwards directly on to the spinal cord, there are immediate signs of major damage:

if it happens in the neck, there may be paralysis, although it may last only a few moments. In American football, the practice of blocking an opponent by a player pushing his head into the opponent's midriff (a move now banned) has caused sudden total paralysis in some instances. Although the player would recover quickly, it was an indication of a potentially dangerous disc herniation. Similar trauma to the neck can occur if there is a blow to the head, for instance in boxing, a fall from a horse, or a car accident. If a major herniation happens in the low back, the victim may notice difficulty with controlling his or her bladder or bowel. This type of injury may need emergency surgery to prevent permanent damage, so the victim should be examined and treated, preferably by a neurosurgeon, as quickly as possible.

If the damaged part of a disc is forced backwards and presses against a nerve root, the result can be pain in the affected area of the back and sometimes referred pain following the nerve pathway into the arm or leg. The disc material acts as a chemical irritant to the tissues it touches, and so causes acute pain. If the nerve root is badly affected, there is not only pain in its pathway, but also signs of neurological damage, such as muscle weakness, tingling or numbness. This condition is usually termed *nerve root compression*, and it is sometimes referred to as a 'trapped nerve'.

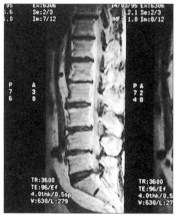

MRI showing a lumbar disc protrusion

Trauma can cause various types of damage to the intervertebral discs. A vertical force, such as a fall on to the bottom, can cause compression injury to the vertebral bones, which can result in bruising or bleeding inside the discs themselves, especially in the middle region of the vertebral column. The discs usually stay in place in these compression injuries, whereas they are very often torn and displaced by injuries which involve bending or twisting movements.

In the low back, disc herniation can happen as a sudden acute episode either during or after activities which usually involve bending and/or twisting movements. Lifting weights incorrectly is a common cause of this type of problem. Very often, the victim feels something 'snap', with immediate sharp pain, and perhaps muscle spasm which pulls the back into a twisted sideways curve (scoliosis). The initial back pain may be accompanied or followed by pain along the nerve pathway into the leg. Simple activities like coughing, sneezing or passing bowel motions may also cause severe pain. Treatment in the early stages may include bed-rest, traction, and pain-relieving and anti-inflammatory drugs. Although most disc injuries happen through a forward bending movement in the spine, disc damage can also occur if any part of the vertebral column is forced backwards into extension, when one or more of the discs can tear and perhaps be pushed forwards.

With age, the intervertebral discs tend to degenerate, changing their composition to a certain extent, and losing their elasticity, which makes them become progressively more rigid. The degeneration processes begin early, sometimes from the late teens onwards, especially in the discs in the neck, which are subjected to a lot of pressure through normal neck movements, especially forward bending. The discs of the low back tend to show degenerative changes later: some deterioration is evident in most people by the age of about thirty. In some cases, the discs become thin centrally, which shows up as a loss of space between the vertebrae on X-ray. This is most common in the lowest spinal joints between L4–L5, and L5–S1, but it can happen at any level in the spine. Occasionally, however, the discs actually gain in thickness by expanding in their central parts in conditions such as osteoporosis.

Degenerative changes do not necessarily cause problems or pain in the discs, but they do make it easier for the disc to become damaged under excessive or abnormal stresses. If the outer area of the annulus fibrosus is damaged, it can cause localized pain in the back or neck without any referred pain, so it may seem similar to pain caused by ligament or muscle injury.

The treatment of most disc problems in the back or neck depends on the circumstances, but in the majority of cases the victim can be successfully treated conservatively, with manual therapy, traction, electrotherapy, or a combination of modalities, and remedial exercises as appropriate. Sometimes injections are used in treatment. If conservative treatment fails, surgery may then be the only option. After any surgery, an accurate rehabilitation programme is essential for full functional recovery.

Facet joint problems

The facet (zygapophyseal) joints formed between the articular processes which lie behind the vertebral bodies can be injured through harsh twisting and bending movements at any level of the spine. Damage can occur in the bones, the cartilage joint surfaces or the soft-tissue structures relating to the joints. The joints can also be affected by wear-and-tear degeneration (osteoarthrosis) or arthritic conditions such as rheumatoid and septic arthritis, or ankylosing spondylitis. Pain stemming from the facet joints is often referred to as 'facet syndrome'.

Treatment is usually conservative, consisting of manual therapy, possibly electrotherapy, and remedial exercises, according to the individual situation.

Fibrositis

Fibrositis is a rather vague name for pain arising from a damaged muscle or tendon. It is often used for conditions where the patient complains of pain and tenderness over a muscular area, when there is no evidence of significant joint involvement or any disease.

In the spine, 'fibrositis' often occurs in the trapezius muscles linking the neck to the shoulder, in the trapezius and rhomboid muscles between the shoulder blades, and in the extensor muscles in the low back. When the practitioner presses on the painful area, there are often very localized tight, 'knotty' areas in the muscles, which are sometimes referred to as 'trigger points'. Treatment directed at the trigger points usually relieves the pain. The treatment may be manual therapy, electrotherapy, or sometimes an injection of local anaesthetic. If the joints close to the affected muscles have become stiff or tender, treatment also has to be directed at them. Remedial exercises are vital for restoring accurate muscle function. The whole process of cure can take quite a long time.

Fractures

Any bone in the spinal column can be broken through trauma, for instance through a fall, a direct blow or a sudden violent shearing movement. In many cases, the bone damage can carry the risk of serious injury to the spinal cord, and treatment is directed at avoiding or minimizing harm in the nervous system. However, a vertebral body can be fractured without jeopardizing the spinal cord, if it is crushed in a *compression* or *wedge* fracture. This type of fracture can also happen from a fall, and usually the impact is taken more or less vertically through the damaged bone. Treatment may consist of a support corset, or the patient may simply be advised not to stress the damaged bone while it is healing, to do remedial exercises under the direction of a physiothera-

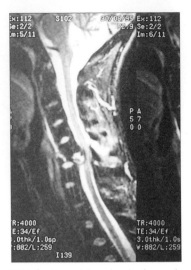

MRI, fracture-dislocation in the neck

pist, and to take care to sit and stand correctly. As soon as the initial pain has subsided, the patient may also be advised to do general exercise, such as gentle swimming. Recovery usually takes about three months, but restoring full function may take longer.

'Kissing' spines

In activities which involve forceful backward bending (hyperextension), such as gymnastics, the spinous processes which form the most prominent parts of the backbone can be pressed together painfully. This can happen through trauma, if the accident has been severe enough to break the anterior longitudinal ligament so that the arches behind the vertebrae are crushed against each other, but this type of accident usually causes damage to several different structures at the same time.

In overuse injury, the spinous processes can be forced against each other on a repetitive basis. Technically this problem has been defined as lumbar interspinous process bursitis, as repeated backward bending can result in a new type of joint forming between the spinous processes. In older people a similar problem can arise because of collapse of the vertebral end-plates, which allows the spinous processes to come too close together during backward movements.

Treatment is usually conservative, using pain-relieving techniques, and mainly concentrating on a remedial exercise programme which strengthens the abdominal and pectoral muscles, and restores body balance through the whole trunk.

Kyphosis

The normal curve of the upper back (thoracic spine) is rounded backwards in what is technically called a kyphosis. An exaggerated kyphosis forms the visible hunchback deformity, and this can happen for a number of reasons.

A child can be born with slightly defective vertebral bodies which develop into the increased curve by the time of adolescence. If the growth points (end-plates) of the vertebral bodies are defective, the front edges of the vertebrae can be eroded, making the vertebrae wedge-shaped as the child goes through adolescence. This causes a marked kyphosis and is called Scheuermann's kyphosis or disease. As the condition usually happens without any known cause, it may also be called idiopathic kyphosis. When necessary, if the curvature is extremely pronounced, a fitted support brace is used to help straighten out the curve, or at least to prevent it from developing any further. The brace may have to be worn overnight, and possibly during the day as well, until the spine has stopped growing. In the worst of cases, corrective surgery may be needed, but it is avoided if at all possible.

In older people an abnormal kyphosis can be caused through a major compression injury, disc degeneration or osteoporosis, all of which can cause loss of height at the front edges of the vertebrae, making them wedge-shaped so that the vertebral column juts backwards abnormally. Treatment depends on the nature of the injury or problem. For pain relief, drugs, mobilization techniques, exercises, or a support brace may all be relevant.

In all cases, however young or old they are, patients have to learn and maintain good postural habits.

Lumbago

Many people use the word 'lumbago' to describe any kind of low back pain. In this sense, lumbago is synonymous with backache. Lumbago has also been more narrowly defined as a sudden acute pain in the low back of the kind which locks the joints into a fixed position. This acute attack usually happens with little provocation. A typical story is that the patient bent down in the normal way to brush his or her teeth, felt a sudden 'click' or stab of pain, and was then unable to straighten up again. The acute pain may last for several days, and is probably best treated with bed-rest, although manipulation may be used successfully in certain cases. Subsequent treatment depends on how the problem develops: if the pain remains acute, there may be a major prolapse of a disc, and surgery may be needed. If the pain subsides, conservative treatment can be continued to help the healing processes. Once recovery is under way, remedial exercises have to be started to regain full mobility and stability in the spinal joints, to help prevent recurrences.

Muscle spasm

An abnormal increase in muscle tone, which makes a muscle become tight and often tender to touch, is called muscle spasm. It can happen for a variety of reasons. When there has been damage in a joint, or a joint has become painful for some reason, the muscle lying over the joint goes into spasm to provide a kind of natural splint for the joint. The tightness in the muscle causes blockage in the normal fibre movement within the muscle and probably reduces the blood flow too, which can cause increasing pain. Muscle tightness can also occur because of stress and viral infections. Sometimes the two go together. The neck is especially vulnerable to spasm from these causes, and spasm in the neck muscles can also cause or aggravate tension headache. Within a whole muscle, certain points can become especially tender, so that they act as focal spots of pain. These are called trigger points, and are common in the neck region (trapezius muscles), along the inner edge of the shoulder blades (trapezius and rhomboids) and lower down the back in the lower parts of the extensor muscles.

Muscle spasm in itself can be reduced by ice applications, hot and cold treatments, massage, and certain forms of electrotherapy. If the muscle spasm is part of a multiple problem, such as some kind of joint injury or derangement, reducing the spasm can be a useful prelude to other types of treatment, such as manipulation or traction. In many cases, the muscle spasm is relieved by accurate treatment of its underlying cause, without specific treatment for the muscle itself. In all cases where muscle function has been impaired, proper muscle balance has to be regained through remedial exercises.

Osteoarthrosis

The alternative names for degeneration in joints are osteoarthrosis and osteoarthritis. In the spine, another term often used is spondylosis (see p.144). The joint surfaces can become roughened, and extra bone can be formed at the edges of the joints, which may even break off in tiny fragments to form loose bodies in a joint. These bony outgrowths are called osteophytes. The degenerative processes are the normal results of wear and tear due to ageing, but they can be late effects from previous injuries, and there can also be a family tendency to osteoarthritic changes in the joints, even though this is not a disease as such.

The signs of degeneration can be picked up on X-rays. People who have done heavy work, such as bricklaying or concrete-breaking using a pneumatic drill, or whose activities have involved repetitive twisting movements, as in an intensive tennis-playing career, are especially likely to have visible signs of joint degeneration in the spine. They may or may not cause pain, and it is perfectly possible to have a severe degree of joint deterioration, but no symptoms.

Treatment is usually conservative, aiming to control pain and maintain the best possible range of joint movement controlled by good muscle function. For acute pain episodes, the joints may be protected for a while in a collar or lumbar support. Manual therapy is usually used, and remedial exercises are vital for restoring and maintaining good physical function.

Piriformis syndrome

The piriformis muscle lies behind the hip joint, and acts to turn the leg outwards into lateral rotation when the hip is straight (extended) and to pull the leg sideways (into abduction) when the hip is bent. Piriformis and the sciatic nerve are very close together, so that any injury to the muscle may put pressure on the sciatic nerve and cause pain and other symptoms through the nerve. When this happens, there is often pain in the low back, especially in the sacroiliac joint region, associated with numbness or tingling in the back of the buttock and thigh. At the extreme of the movement, it can be painful to turn the hip on the affected side both outwards and inwards. There may be pain on lifting the leg straight upwards in the straight-leg-raising test, and tests for the sacroiliac joint may also be positive.

Treatment usually consists of physiotherapy, including stretching for the piriformis, manual therapy, possibly ultrasound or other electrotherapy techniques, and remedial exercises. If conservative treatment fails, more invasive measures such as surgery may be used as a last resort.

Sacroiliac joint problems

The sacroiliac joint can be strained by a bending and twisting movement. Although the joint structures are extremely strong, the joint becomes more vulnerable to strain if the ligaments are loosened or weakened by hormonal changes in women, or undermined by any of the various diseases and arthritic conditions which can affect the joint, such as, for instance, ankylosing spondylitis, rheumatoid arthritis, gout and Paget's disease.

Even a strong, normal sacroiliac joint can suffer a shearing strain if you bend and turn, for instance, to put a heavy case into the boot of a car. Tennis, squash and golf cause particular pressures over the joint, and the hip joint is often affected as well. Once one sacroiliac joint has been injured, it is not uncommon for the related joints of the pelvis to become involved, so that you may notice pain in the sacroiliac joint of the other side, in either or both hips, in the pubic region, and radiating into the groin(s).

Pain from the sacroiliac joint is generally felt directly over the joint in the lowest part of the back. It can become especially sore if you have to stand and bend forwards slightly in your work, as teachers often have to do, or if you have to sit in a chair which is not properly supportive, for instance a badly designed swivel chair with an unstable backrest.

Treatment for sacroiliac joint injury is usually conservative, and may consist of manual therapy, possibly electrotherapy, and remedial exercises, as appropriate.

Scheuermann's disease

Disturbance in the growth areas (end-plates) of the vertebral bodies, which is technically called epiphysitis, can lead to erosions and visible defects in the front edges of the bones, causing wedging. The technical term for the bone defects is osteochondritis or osteochondrosis. Schmorl's nodes may also appear: these are protrusions of material from the nucleus of an adjoining disc, which press into the vertebral body and gradually erode the bone. When the node is in the central region of the bone, it is usually painless, but if it appears towards the front edge of the bone it can contribute to the collapse of the bone and consequent wedging.

Scheuermann's disease happens most commonly in adolescent males between the ages of twelve and eighteen, and mainly affects the lower thoracic vertebrae in the central region of the spine. The cause is not known, although it is often associated with an abnormally rich blood supply in the end-plate. It is thought that excessive loading, especially through sport, may be a major causative factor.

The condition may happen without necessarily causing pain, but if it is painful the patient usually has to rest from any activities involving heavy loading or pain-provoking movements. In very bad cases, a brace may be fitted to protect the joints and prevent deterioration in the shape of the spine. Remedial exercises can help to improve function, although any deformity cannot usually be reversed. Good postural habits must be instilled and maintained. Sometimes the condition can be an underlying cause in back pain later on, even though it caused the patient no problems as a teenager.

Sciatica

Pain radiating along the course of the sciatic nerve, down the back of the leg into the calf is properly termed sciatica. The name is also often misused as a label for referred pain affecting the buttock or other parts of the leg, although such referred pain usually stems from other nerve roots. The symptoms can vary from extreme pain to only a slight disturbance of the sensations in the leg. They may be constant if there is severe compression of the nerve root, perhaps due to a massive disc herniation, or the symptoms may only come on when you sit or stand in a certain position.

The exact cause of sciatica is not fully understood, as it is possible to have a large disc protrusion taking up space in the spinal canal without necessarily having any referred pain or symptoms.

Treatment varies according to the situation. It may be bedrest, protection in a firm or soft lumbar corset, manual therapy, traction or surgery. Remedial exercises are generally restricted or avoided while the referred symptoms are present, although they are usually introduced gradually during the recovery phases.

Scoliosis

Scoliosis is the technical name for an abnormal sideways twist (lateral curvature) in the spinal column. In adults, a scoliosis can develop suddenly as the result of injury which makes the back lock with acute muscle spasm on one side. This type of scoliosis usually disappears once treatment has removed the cause of the spasm. It is common for adults to have at least some degree of scoliosis if they have taken part in sports which involve intensive twisting and bending of the spine, such as rowing and tennis. In most cases, this type of scoliosis does not of itself cause pain, and it is only noticeable on certain movements of the spine.

In children and adolescents, a marked scoliosis can develop and cause serious problems, partly because it creates a visible deformity or hunchback, and partly because a severe scoliosis which affects the upper back can interfere with the person's breathing. The scoliosis can be congenital, caused because the child was born with defects in the structure of the spinal bones. If it develops later, it happens apparently spontaneously, and is called idiopathic scoliosis. This happens most commonly in young teenagers, especially girls, just at the onset of puberty. As the youngster grows, the scoliosis can get much worse.

There are various ways of treating this problem. If the scoliosis is only mild when it is first seen, the paediatric orthopaedic specialist may choose simply to keep it under observation by checking on the child every few months. If it is bad enough, a special support brace for the spine is fitted, which the child is expected to wear for up to twenty-two hours per day. Electrical muscle stimulation to help correct the muscle balance controlling the spinal joints may be tried as an alternative to bracing in mild or moderate cases, and this is usually done by using a small machine which can be applied for several hours at a time, often overnight. This regime should be backed with a strict remedial exercise programme. In all cases, the child is encouraged to be active, and to participate in all possible sports apart from contact sports or those requiring extreme body movements, such as trampolining and competitive gymnastics. In the worst of cases, surgery may be needed if the scoliosis progresses beyond a certain limit. This is of course a major procedure, after which full recovery to normal activities takes at least six months or longer.

Short leg syndrome

A slight difference in leg lengths is common in most people. However, leg length inequality can contribute to low back pain, and in some cases is a major factor. When one leg is relatively short, the pelvis usually tilts to compensate, and this can cause a minor scoliosis in the spine. Pain associated with leg length discrepancy, which affects one side of the low back, usually happens on the side of the longer leg, although it is not fully understood why this should be so.

In order to identify whether a visible leg length difference is due to differences in bone length ('real shortening') or due to tilting of the pelvis ('apparent shortening') the practitioner measures the distance from the outer part of the hip to the inner side of the ankle, from the front tip of the pelvic bone (anterior superior iliac spine) to the inner ankle, and from the tip of the breast-bone (xiphisternum) to the inner ankle.

If your pain is directly linked to the leg length difference, you are likely to feel it most when you are standing or walking, and it should be relieved, at least to a certain extent, if you use a raise in your shoe. If it makes a real difference, you may benefit from having your day shoes built up to the appropriate height. However, do not rush into expensive alterations, as they may prove to be unnecessary if your problem is only temporary, and can be resolved with treatment and remedial exercises.

Spinal cord injury

This type of accident can happen through a fall from a height, especially if you land awkwardly and twist your back or neck as you hit the ground. Some of the common causes of these accidents are horse-riding falls, parachutes which fail to open, car accidents at speed, and diving into shallow water. Once the spinal cord is broken, it cannot mend itself (regenerate), so the injury results in a degree of paralysis which affects the area below the level of the fracture.

If the spinal cord is completely severed, the paralysis is total, and the victim cannot move the affected area, which also loses all its normal feelings. Because of the loss of sensation and the reduction in the normal blood flow in the paralysed parts, the patient's skin becomes vulnerable to pressure sores, which can become dangerous if they get infected. Looking after the skin by moving as much and as often as possible in the wheelchair is a necessary routine in the patient's everyday life. This is a priority for carers looking after the quadriplegic patient who cannot lift his or her bodyweight off the chair to relieve the pressure. Once an area of skin has broken down, the patient usually has to spend time in bed so that the wound can heal without further pressure being exerted on it.

If the patient's paralysis is partial, the disability may vary from severe to not too bad. Over time, the victim may gradually recover more movement and sensation. It may be possible to walk with crutches if the paralysis is not complete or if the damage is not at too high a level of the spinal cord. Otherwise, the patient is confined to a wheelchair. Depending on the individual, driving, sports activities and work are all possible for the wheelchair-bound patient. Even in complete paralysis from the neck down, it can still be possible to control a wheelchair using a special lever operated by the mouth. Similar devices can be set up to work switches, catches and machines in the home, so the disabled person can lead a reasonably full life with at least an element of independence.

Spinal stenosis

When there is narrowing in the space behind the vertebral bodies (the spinal canal), it can cause pressure on the spinal nerves, especially the nerve roots. The narrowing may affect the central part of the canal or the openings to either side through which the nerve roots pass. The problem tends to occur in the low back only, not the upper back or neck. It causes back pain together with symptoms in the legs which may be pain, numbness, tingling or weakness, or a combination of these at different times. A typical feature is pain due to standing upright or walking which can be relieved by resting or by bending forward.

Many factors may be involved in causing spinal stenosis. It can be a congenital feature which you are born with, so that the symptoms come on very early. The problem can also develop in later life as the result of a genetic tendency which has influenced the structure of the spinal canal. More often, the problem develops through degenerative changes in one or more discs and the nearby facet joints. The majority of patients with spinal stenosis are over 60 years old. Spinal stenosis can also be associated with traumatic injury, surgery which has failed, or various diseases which cause disruption to the spinal bones.

Once diagnosed, the problem may be treated by protecting the area while the pain is acute, either with bed-rest or a corset. As quickly as possible, painless exercise is encouraged. Apart from localized exercises, riding a bicycle may be the best form of aerobic exercise for the patient. As a means of transport, it is a good alternative to walking. If conservative treatment fails, surgery is usually considered.

Spondylolisthesis

When one vertebral body slips forward relative to another, the technical name for the bone slippage is spondylolisthesis. It happens because the vertebrae become unstable, very often due to spondylolysis or stress fractures in the vertebral arches behind the vertebral bodies. It can also happen because of severe degeneration in the spinal joints which leads to instability. This problem occurs most commonly at the lowest levels of the spine, but it can also happen slightly higher up. Like spondylolysis, it tends to happen to sports players such as cricketers, rowers and gymnasts who twist, bend and possibly overload their spine, especially through repetitive training.

The symptoms of spondylolisthesis may be quite mild, even when the displacement is large, but the injury can also cause severe pain, with or without referred symptoms into the legs. The pain is usually only related to activity, and may

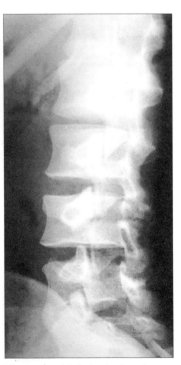

X-ray, spondylolisthesis, showing the defect in the pars interarticularis

only come on after the sports activity which has caused the damage.

Diagnosis is usually made on the basis of the history of pain and X-rays which show the bone displacement. Treatment is generally conservative, ranging from bed-rest or immobilization in a plaster cast for a very severe case in a young person, to pain-relieving techniques combined with rest from any pain-causing activities probably for a period of three to six months. Remedial exercises are essential for restoring stability. The return to sport has to be very gradual, and should always be combined with a comprehensive fitness programme for good body balance.

Spondylolysis

A defect in the strut of bone (pars interarticularis) which links the superior and inferior articular facets in the bony arch behind a vertebra is called a spondylolysis. It is effectively a crack, which can form a weak point in the bone, although it does not necessarily cause pain. It is not always certain why it happens, and it is sometimes picked up on X-rays incidentally, without being linked to any particular problem. Hereditary factors may play a part, and there may be a congenital weakness in the bone structure. However, in many cases the spondylolysis is a fracture caused by trauma or repetitive stresses.

The traumatic fracture can happen through a direct blow to the side of the spine, perhaps from rough tackling in rugby or American football, or a hard kick in contact karate. A bone crack due to repetitive stresses is called a stress or fatigue fracture. It can be caused by repeated twisting movements under load, for example through intensive practice bowling in cricket, diving, tumbling routines in gymnastics, rowing and javelin throwing.

Spondylolysis occurs in patients of all ages, and is found in children as young as 6. It usually occurs in the low back (lumbar spine) or lower part of the upper back (thoracic spine). If it causes pain, this can be severe at times, although it may only become bad after prolonged activity. There may be spasm in the muscles lying over the injured area. The pain may be localized to the affected area of the spine, or it may radiate down into the buttock or leg on the same side.

Diagnosis is usually made on the basis of the pain pattern and the presence of the bone defect, which may show up best on X-rays taken at an angle to the spine (oblique views).

Treatment is usually conservative, consisting of pain-relieving therapy and remedial exercises. Full recovery usually occurs and the patient should return to all sporting activities, even though the bone defect may not mend, so that it remains visible on X-rays.

Spondylosis

Degeneration due to wear-and-tear and perhaps the long-term effects of injury in the spinal joints is often referred to as spondylosis, which can be used as a synonym for osteoarthritis or osteoarthrosis. The name covers a great many different degenerative effects, such as the formation of bony outgrowths (osteophytes) on the edges of the vertebral bodies, disruption in the position and movements of related facet joints, and degeneration of the intervertebral discs. Such problems can occur anywhere in the vertebral column, but are especially common in the neck and low back, where they are referred to as cervical and lumbar spondylosis respectively.

When pain arises, treatment may consist of rest from painful activities, pain-relieving drugs, support from an elastic lumbar corset or a soft collar for the neck, manual therapy, possibly electrotherapy, and remedial exercises once the acute phase has passed. If the patient is overweight, weight reduction through increased general exercise and diet control will also certainly be recommended.

Torticollis

If the neck becomes fixed in a twisted and bent position, the technical term is torticollis, but the problem is also referred to as 'wry neck', or in milder cases as a 'crick' in the neck. The head is usually bent to one side and may be turned to the opposite side. The problem can be congenital, when the baby is born with one of the neck muscles relatively shortened (in a contracture). Treatment simply consists of stretching the muscle gently to loosen it and correct the head position.

The problem can arise in both children and adults through viral infection, when the neck becomes very stiff and painful. Sometimes the cause is not obvious, although the neck problem may coincide with other symptoms such as a sore throat or ear ache. It eases spontaneously with due rest. In adolescents and adults torticollis can arise as the result of an injury. When the stiffness and deformity come on suddenly without warning, for instance on waking in the morning, or on slightly turning the head, the problem can be purely mechanical, or perhaps a mixture of mechanical and viral factors. Any tissue damage, including a bone fracture, muscle tear, ligament strain or disc injury can cause torticollis. Treatment depends on the situation, but generally consists of pain-relieving measures including manual therapy, and perhaps protection in a soft collar. Once the acute phase has passed, remedial exercises are usually started.

Vertebral artery insufficiency

Because the vertebral arteries are protected within the bone structure of the neck (cervical) vertebrae, they can also suffer interference if there is injury or degeneration in the structures of the vertebrae. Typical symptoms include feelings of dizziness or fainting when the head is tilted into a certain position, and the problem may also contribute to headaches.

There has to be careful diagnosis, to exclude other possible causes of similar symptoms, and to identify whether in fact you might have more than one problem. Treatment is usually conservative, consisting of gentle manual therapy to improve the joint function, remedial exercises for the joints, and often special exercises to improve your balance mechanisms.

Whiplash

The most common cause of a whiplash injury is a car accident, in which the victim is jolted by a severe force from a vehicle behind. As the car is shunted forwards, the victim's head is thrown first backwards, then forcibly forwards as the car comes to a halt. The force can damage the neck bones, ligaments, discs, muscles or a combination of tissues. Although seat belts and head restraints have reduced the distance through which the head can be thrown, the trauma to the neck from even a minor shunting injury usually causes intense and long-lasting pain, together with neck stiffness. Immediately after this type of accident, even if it might seem only minor, the victim should be examined in the hospital casualty department to exclude brain injury or bone fracture. In the initial recovery stages, the neck is usually protected in a firm or soft collar, according to how much support is needed to provide some relief of pain. If any treatment is given, it is usually limited to very gentle manual therapy.

The severe pain can last up to three months or more before it gradually starts to abate. Once the pain is less intense, treatment can be extended, and electrical muscle stimulation may be used to revive efficient function in the spinal muscles. Gentle remedial exercises may also start at this stage, although any kind of normal sport is usually still out of the question. It may take six months or longer to be able to re-start even relatively gentle sporting activities, and full recovery generally takes at least a year.

INFLAMMATORY AND METABOLIC DISEASES

There are innumerable conditions and diseases which can cause or contribute to spinal pain. Inflammatory conditions include Reiters disease, psoriatic arthritis, and inflammatory bowel disorders such as ulcerative colitis. Probably the most common of the inflammatory conditions are ankylosing spondylitis and rheumatoid arthritis. Metabolic diseases can affect the body's bones in conditions such as Paget's disease, osteomalacia and hyperparathyroidism. Joints can also be affected, for instance in gout, which usually affects peripheral joints such as those of the toes, ankles, hands or knees. Osteoporosis, which is considered to be a metabolic disease, is probably one of the most common of these conditions.

Ankylosing spondylitis

Ankylosing spondylitis is a rheumatic condition which can cause pain and progressive stiffness throughout the back. It usually starts in a sacroiliac joint and spreads up through the spinal joints, eventually affecting the shoulders, rib cage joints and arms. The hips and leg joints can also become involved. The joints affected usually become painful at first, and then gradually seize up until they are almost completely immobile. Once it is well advanced, the condition can cause considerable deformity, especially if the upper back and neck are badly affected, when the patient develops a severe hunchback which makes it difficult to lift the head up at all.

Pain tends to happen in episodes, even though the condition is a developing process, so it can seem just like musculoskeletal back pain caused by injury or poor posture. Sometimes the patient also feels unwell during an acute phase, although this may seem simply the result of extreme pain. A typical feature of the pain is early morning stiffness. Very often, there are other symptoms too, such as plantar fasciitis, which causes pain and spasm under the sole of the

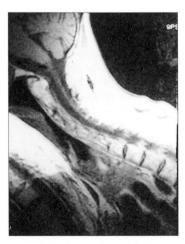

MRI, ankylosing spondylitis in the neck

foot, and uviitis, which causes painful inflammation in the eye. These may or may not coincide with the episodes of back pain.

The first signs of ankylosing spondylitis usually show during the teen years, although they may come on earlier or later. Males seem to be affected more than females. There may be a hereditary factor, and it is not uncommon to find that some relative to the victim also suffers from the condition. On blood tests, the antigen HLA-B27 is usually found, although this antigen can be present in the blood of people who are not affected by the condition. As the condition advances, X-rays show typical changes as the joint linkages seize up.

Apart from some pain relief, there is little if any effective medical or surgical treatment for this condition. However, a regular programme of all-round rehabilitation exercises for the whole body is known to help stop the progressive stiffening of the joints, keeping the body in working order. One of my patients came to me in his early forties, having suffered from ankylosing spondylitis for twenty years. He had to take painkillers every day, and his posture was extremely poor. He was a heavy smoker, and this was impairing his lung function, which was gradually also being undermined by stiffening in the rib cage. With great reluctance, he was persuaded to start working out twice a week, using the Norsk Sequence-Training rehabilitation equipment. His motivation increased when he realized after about six weeks that he no longer needed regular painkillers, and people began to remark on the improvement in his posture. For the last ten years, he has maintained a regular training regime, and so has been able to live a full and active life.

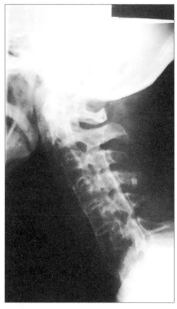

X-ray, showing the effects of ankylosing spondylitis in the neck

Osteoporosis

Osteoporosis can happen for a variety of reasons, including as a result of certain diseases and cancers. However, it occurs most often through the effects of ageing. With increasing age, the body's bones can lose their ability to absorb shock and support loads. There may be a loss of normal bone density, which shows up if a bone scan is taken. Any bones can be affected by osteoporosis, and the bone scan reveals areas which are particularly vulnerable. The problem can happen in men, but it is more common in women, especially through the effects of the menopause. The risk is also increased if there is a history of osteoporosis in the family.

Osteoporosis may be present without causing symptoms, but it means that the affected bones are brittle and therefore likely to break even under relatively slight pressure, knocks or trauma. The neck of the thigh bone (femur) is a common site of osteoporosis, and as it is an important weightbearing bone, breaking it is a major injury. Osteoporosis in the spine causes gradual collapse of the vertebral bodies, so that the victim gradually loses height and gets shorter. A typical feature is the hunchback appearance due to increased curvature (kyphosis) in the upper back, which is often referred to as the 'dowager's hump'. Apart from the increased risk of fractures, osteoporosis can cause pain.

Prevention depends on an adequate intake and absorption of calcium through the diet. If in doubt as to the best way of increasing calcium input, the patient should be referred to a dietician for specific advice. Hormone Replacement Therapy (HRT) can help to protect females going through the menopause from osteoporosis. One of the most important preventive factors is regular exercise, and it has been shown that even in the very old, bone density can be improved through general physical activity. It is also the case that the old person is less likely to fall over if he or she has maintained good muscle strength and co-ordination through well-balanced exercises.

Treatment for osteoporotic pain consists of controlled and progressive active exercises to improve the bone condition. Electrical muscle stimulation may be used in certain cases. Full-thrust manipulations are contra-indicated because of the high risk of damaging the fragile bones.

Rheumatoid arthritis

Rheumatoid arthritis is an inflammatory condition which most often affects the synovial joints of the hands, feet, elbows and knees, but it can also affect any other synovial joint, including the spinal facet joints at any level from the low back to the neck. If the disease progresses, it causes a gradual deterioration of the affected joint, with painful swelling and deformity in most cases. The cause is not certain, but a hereditary factor is often involved, and it is common to find that a close relative has also had the problem.

The disease is usually treated with medicines and spells of physiotherapy to maintain muscle tone and strength. When the disease is in an active phase, exercises cannot be done, as they are too painful, and the patient often feels quite ill. Rest is the best way of controlling an acute episode. If the joints of the hands, feet or knees become particularly painful, there may be a case for replacing them surgically with artificial joints. Sometimes the disease 'burns out', so that the joint degeneration does not progress beyond a certain point.

INFECTIONS, ILLNESSES AND VIRUSES

Infections can affect the spinal structures, causing intense pain which is not directly related to movement, and which remains fairly constant most of the time. These infections include infective discitis (inflammation in the intervertebral disc) and osteomyelitis (bone infection), which can occur even in very young children. The child usually complains of searing pain in the back or referred into the abdominal region, hips or legs, which may make it difficult to sit down or walk around, although the pain is usually also present when the child lies down. Usually the child has a high temperature, which may have been present before the pain started. Basic blood tests usually prove that infection is present, and MRI or CT scans may confirm what the infection is. Such illnesses in patients of any age have to be treated promptly and accurately with appropriate antibiotics, according to the situation.

Tuberculosis

Tuberculosis is a disease which primarily affects the lungs, but as tuberculous arthritis it can cause joint pain and damage, usually in the arm or leg joints, but also in the back, especially the sacroiliac joints or the intervertebral discs and bones of the lumbar spine. As in other forms of septic arthritis, which can be caused by a variety of different organisms, the disease attacks the affected joints, causing progressive and sometimes dramatic structural disruption if the process is not halted by immediate accurate treatment, especially appropriate antibiotics.

Many other illnesses and diseases can cause symptoms relating to the spinal joints without necessarily causing tissue damage as such.

Bronchitis and pleurisy

Bronchitis and pleurisy are chest illnesses which can cause pain around the chest wall which affects the thoracic spine (upper back). These illnesses can also refer pain elsewhere: for instance, some types of pleurisy, which is inflammation in the lining of the lung, can cause severe pain in the left trapezius muscle and side of the neck, and this can seem exactly like pain from a mechanical injury.

Shingles

Shingles is an infection which causes severe pain along the pathway of a nerve. It very often affects the chest wall, and sometimes the radiating pain is the first sign, followed later by the tell-tale line of red spots. Another typical pattern of the shingles rash follows one side of the neck and runs up over the head, often into the eye on the same side. There can be a gap of several days between the onset of the apparent spinal or radiating pain and the appearance of the spots. One very unusual case was that of the 37-year-old lady I treated who had had several skiing accidents involving her neck and shoulders. I started treating her three months after she had suffered a bad fall on to the back of her head, which had resulted in severe neck stiffness. She had suffered no head injury, although one eye flickered constantly following the accident. Her main complaint was of neck pain, coupled with variable pain in either shoulder, and pain alternating with pins and needles in both her arms.

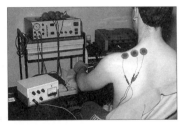

Biofeedback to relax the trapezius muscle

The symptoms improved with twice-weekly treatment including neck traction, mobilizations, biofeedback(see p.114) to help reduce the tension in the trapezius muscles, and remedial exercises for the spine, shoulders and arms. During this period, although she had to wear a soft collar most of the time, the patient managed to continue her work as a secretary, as well as frequently playing squash and going on sailing trips. However, after one month, the pain affecting the neck intensified, although it was variable. The eye flickering stopped, but, curiously, about ten days later the patient developed a severe eye infection, which was initially diagnosed as conjunctivitis. When the eye failed to respond to treatment, the patient consulted a specialist, who identified shingles, and sure enough some days later the rash appeared from the neck over the head and into the upper part of the face. After a prolonged period of rest, the patient recovered. Although her eye did not regain full vision, her neck became virtually painfree.

Myalgic encephalomyelitis (ME)

Myalgic encephalomyelitis (ME) is a relatively new disease in Britain, and is the subject of continuing research. It may have several forms, although patients with differing symptoms are usually diagnosed as having ME on the basis of a battery of blood tests, including one to show whether the VP1 antigen is present. The common factors among patients are severe, disabling fatigue, linked with long-standing infections, such as chesty coughs and sore throats. ME patients often suffer from depression, and body aching which affects either the muscles or the joints or sometimes both. Physiotherapy care for ME patients involves trying to reduce any musculoskeletal pains, and helping them to increase their ability to exercise, which is usually very limited at first. Their overall care involves teamwork, usually between a neurological consultant, general practitioner, homeopath, physiotherapist, psychologist, sometimes a social worker, possibly an osteopath, and very often complementary practitioners such as an acupuncturist, reflexologist and aromatherapist.

Glandular fever

Glandular fever is another debilitating illness which can strike active and supposedly healthy young people. It is relatively common among teenagers and university students, but can occur at any age. Typically, it can cause pain and stiffness in the neck where the glands are swollen and inflamed, but it can also be an underlying factor in pain felt elsewhere in the spine. For example, a marathon runner, G., aged 29, whose job involved extensive travelling, was preparing for the Olympic trials. Over the space of two months he had built up his training to one hundred miles per week. He had been maintaining this training load for three weeks when he ran into trouble. One winter morning on a normal training run he felt a sudden sharp pain in his left side, all the way round his lower rib cage from the spine in the central area of his back. He had run five miles, and he jogged the one mile home. In the afternoon, he ran three miles very fast, and experienced extremely severe pain in his left side as he ran downhill.

He felt so stiff that he lay down for the whole of the next day, and felt better. The morning after that he noticed some sharp shooting pains in his left side on waking up, but they eased, so he went out for a ten-mile run that evening and a six-mile run the next morning. Later that day he came to me for physiotherapy treatment, convinced that in some way he had strained the middle region of his back. He had a previous history of left-sided low back pain, but had never suffered from problems in the middle back region.

In fact, from the history and physical examination there was no biomechanical explanation for G.'s left-sided trunk pain, even though there was localized tenderness to the left side of his thoracic spine. On the other hand, he had the symptoms of some kind of infection, as he had noticed pain in breathing during the night, he had slept badly since the pain came on, and he felt that a 'cold' had come on two days later, after he had done the ten-mile run. G. was therefore referred to a consultant physician, who did several blood tests, and diagnosed glandular fever three weeks later, by which time G. was feeling a lot better. About a week after that, G. re-started running and rapidly built up to one hundred miles a week again. Although he was obviously impatiently keen to feel fully fit for the Olympic trials, he exercised caution in checking his early-morning (basal) pulse, using the guideline that if it was raised above the normal average by ten beats or more, he would not train that day.

G. managed to keep up his training schedule without major setbacks until the trials, but sadly failed to gain a place in the Olympic team. On the positive side, however, he has continued to enjoy his running over many years since then. His case was unusual, in that recovery from glandular fever is usually a very slow process, and victims often need several years before they can build up to really intensive physical exercise regimes again.

Spinal conditions: how to cope

- Don't attempt to diagnose your own problem
- Don't worry unduly about your condition
- Don't consult several practitioners at once
- Don't interpret and alter instructions
- Do think positively
- Do follow through your treatment and self-help regimes
- Do ask your practitioner for guidance if you have doubts
- Do ask for a second opinion if treatment fails

Exercise tests

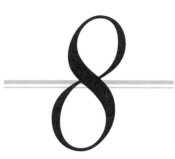

FUNCTIONAL TESTING

When practitioners do biomechanical tests to assess how well your trunk and limbs are working, we do not set absolute standards. In a healthy person, the body's joints can move in certain directions and not in others. To this extent, basic joint movements are standardized. But individuals vary enormously according to various factors, including inherited bone and muscle (skeletal) structure, patterns of activities and sports, postural habits, growth phases, and the effects of ageing. Your ability to perform functional tests can also alter according to the time of day, your eating and drinking patterns, and your emotional and physical state. You are likely to perform best when you are feeling fit, healthy and fresh, worst when you are especially tired or stressed physically and/or emotionally.

Specialized isokinetic testing equipment is a sophisticated way of measuring your physical capacities and joint movements. It is becoming increasingly important in medico-legal cases, where scientific precision is important for establishing how much spinal damage has happened following a car crash or accident at work, or whether the victim is in fact exaggerating the amount of functional impairment he or she has suffered from a back injury.

For most general purposes, however, monitoring can be done efficiently through a battery of movement tests. Accuracy is best achieved if the same person does the original testing and any subsequent tests, although it is possible for different practitioners to do the follow-up if the parameters

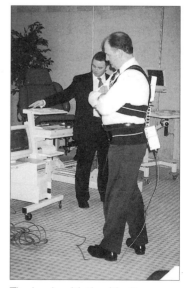

The Lumbar Motion Monitor (Chattanooga), computerized equipment for measuring spinal movement

are strictly defined. To a certain extent it is also possible for you to do the simple biomechanical tests on your own, or with a partner where necessary, without involving a practitioner. A sports coach or physical education teacher should easily be able to set up the tests and apply them.

Any battery of exercise tests is designed to find out how well you can do each specified movement, whether there are any movements which you simply cannot do, and whether any movement causes you pain. If you do experience pain, you must tell the practitioner straight away. In general, you should always try to avoid pain, so never try to do exercises or movements which you know bring on or increase your spinal pain.

The exercises described here are my personal choice for a comprehensive programme of remedial and protective exercises for the trunk, and for functional assessment of sports players. Depending on each individual case, I employ a selection of the test-exercises. Having assessed the person's strengths and weaknesses, and found out if any of the movements is too difficult or too easy to be included, I then construct a personal programme with special emphasis on areas of weakness, tightness or relative incoordination. The remedial exercise programme may also include other exercises which I have not used as tests, but which are included because they are relevant to the patient's injury or sport.

The tests are repeated at intervals to check whether functional improvements are being made. Re-testing is not only a useful guide to progress; it also serves to motivate patients to persevere with their remedial exercise programmes. Re-testing can take place at one- two- or three-monthly intervals. The timing can vary according to convenience. Some patients prefer to come for re-testing sooner and more frequently, in order to maintain motivation. Others might be confident that they will be disciplined in keeping to the exercise programme, and so may only need testing rarely, to assess whether the programme should be extended with more advanced exercises or to decide whether the patient is fit for a full return to normal sporting activities.

THE REMEDIAL EXERCISE PROGRAMME

The remedial exercises are geared to help restore full function after spinal problems, and to prevent a recurrence of pain, stiffness, weakness or movement limitation. Movements for the arms and legs are included, as your limbs exert an influence on your spine, and equally protect your spine from undue stresses if they work properly. The exercises combine basic flexibility with strength and co-ordination.

The exercises should be done very precisely, without any strain. The photographs illustrating each of the test-exercises given below show exactly how they should be done. If you find any of the exercises difficult, you should do only a few repetitions at a time, making sure that the movements are performed absolutely correctly. If you have an area which is especially weak or tight, you must concentrate on improving it. Do not just do those exercises which you find easiest. In a remedial exercise programme, the exercises you find easiest should be done least, while you build up your capacity for the movements which are harder.

Active sports players and athletes often make the mistake of thinking that they should feel a strain or reaction during the exercises, if they are to gain anything from them. This is not so. On the contrary, you should feel no immediate effect. The old saying 'no gain without pain' is debatable in any context. With remedial exercises, any reaction is likely to aggravate existing back pain or even cause stiffness or injury. If a movement causes pain during or after its execution, it also causes muscle inhibition, and your attempts at exercises then become counter-productive. If anything, if you do the exercises correctly and progressively, you should feel that you have not made enough effort. Any feeling of strain is likely to make the exercise a waste of time.

> With remedial exercises you only gain *without* pain

The long-term aim of the remedial exercises is to establish a good balance between mobility and stability through the whole body in general, and within the spinal joints in particular. Like a physical fitness programme, your remedial exercise programme should be progressive, so that you build up the amount you can do in easy stages. Once you are back to full fitness after a back problem, you should maintain a balanced regime of exercises as a background to your other training or physical activities. Your maintenance programme may be less than the final stage of the recovery programme, but it should be consistent.

The far-sighted sports player who has never had a back problem should do a combination of at least some of these exercises as an injury prevention programme within an overall training schedule. The exercises are also suitable for general keep-fit purposes and body conditioning, even if you are not training specifically for a sport. Do remember that it takes about three months for muscles to adapt to a muscle training programme, so you need to maintain your schedule as a regular routine for at least that long, and preferably indefinitely as a long-term daily fitness routine.

Warning

- Never do exercises against your doctor's advice, especially if you have medical problems such as high blood pressure
- If in doubt, check with your doctor before embarking on any kind of training or remedial exercise programme
- Never do exercises or movements which cause pain either while you are doing them or afterwards
- If a particular exercise causes pain one day, even though you have been able to do it comfortably before, leave it out for a couple of days, and reintroduce it gradually when it causes no pain
- If in doubt, always be guided by a qualified practitioner

Test-exercises

1. The bent-knee sit-up, feet unsupported (in the crook-lying, or hook-lying position)

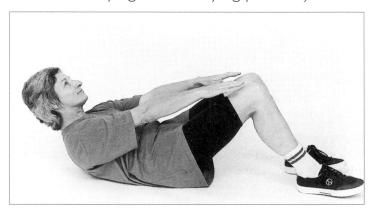

Lying on your back with your knees bent, feet flat on the floor and not fixed or held, hold your arms straight out in front of you, and sit up to reach towards your knees with your hands, keeping your head and neck in line with your trunk. Slowly lower yourself down, uncurling from the lower back, and relax.

Precautions

Do not bring your head forward or strain your neck to try to make the movement easier. Do not sit right up or take your hands past your knees. Do not do the movement if it causes pain.

Effects

This is a co-ordination exercise which also strengthens the abdominal muscles concentrically as you lift the weight of your trunk, head and arms up against gravity, and eccentrically as you reverse the movement. It co-ordinates the action of the muscles in front of and behind your pelvis because you have to stabilize your legs using your gluteal muscles and hamstrings at the same time as you activate the abdominals to sit up. You may find it difficult to do because your feet tend to lift off the floor, even if your abdominal muscles are reasonably strong and you can easily achieve test-exercise 3. What this means is that your co-ordination is poor and needs to be improved.

If you cannot achieve the co-ordination movement, you are more likely to be vulnerable to episodes of backache or acute pain. This is true even if your abdominal muscles are strong in themselves. If you suffer an acute episode of low back pain, you may lose the ability to perform the movement, even if you could do it easily before, but it returns as your back gets better.

As a test

1 Can you do the movement correctly without pain?
2 If you can achieve the movement, time yourself over one minute and count the number of repetitions you achieve.
3 If you cannot, you should try exercise 3, and leave out exercise 2.

As an exercise

Start with five repetitions, if the exercise is difficult at first. Build up to five sets of ten repetitions.

2. The bent-knee sit-up, feet free, elbows to knees

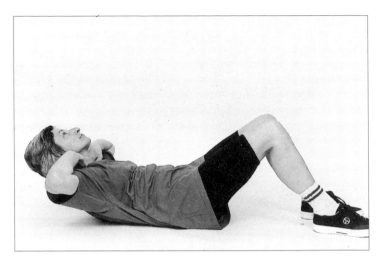

Lie on your back with your knees bent, feet flat on the floor and not fixed, hands on either side of your neck; sit up, being careful to keep your arms, head and neck in line with your trunk. Slowly uncurl to lower your trunk and head back to the floor, then relax.

Precautions
Do not strain your head and neck to perform the movement. Do not sit right up to bring your chest close to your thighs. Do not work through pain.

Effects
This is an advanced version of exercise 1. If you can do it efficiently, you have excellent co-ordination around your trunk, pelvis and lower back, as well as good concentric and eccentric strength in your abdominal muscles.

As a test
Count the number of repetitions you can perform accurately over one minute.

As an exercise
Start with five repetitions; build up to three sets of ten repetitions.

3. The bent-knee sit-up, feet fixed

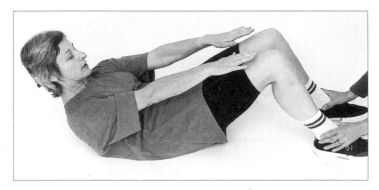

Lying on your back, with knees bent and feet fixed under a block or held by a partner, and keeping your arms straight, sit up to reach towards your knees with your hands. Slowly lower back to the floor and relax.

Precautions
As for exercises 1 and 2.

Effects
This is a movement to improve the tone in your abdominal muscles. You strengthen them concentrically by lifting the weight of your trunk, head and arms against gravity, and eccentrically as you reverse the movement with control. Poor abdominals leave the trunk virtually unsupported and make it difficult for you to maintain good posture while sitting or standing, and impossible for you to lift even light weights safely. If you find the exercise difficult, it is vital to practise the movement frequently, although you must avoid pain, so you may only be able to do a very limited range. If you cannot do the movement at all because of pain or inhibition, you need to work on a special programme to improve your abdominal muscle tone before working on functional strength (see pp.116–17).

Without basic abdominal strength, you cannot hope to have the necessary co-ordination to perform exercises 1 and 2 properly.

As a test
1 Can you perform the movement properly, at all, with or without pain?
2 If you can do the exercise without pain, count the number of repetitions you can achieve in one minute.

As an exercise
Start with five repetitions; build up to five sets of ten repetitions.

4. The twist sit-up with knees bent, feet fixed

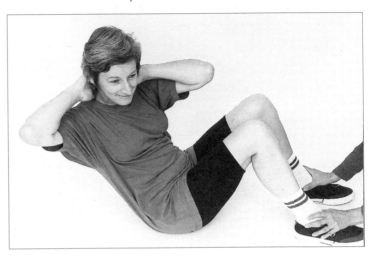

Lying on your back with your feet fixed or held, hands behind your neck and elbows held back level with your head, sit up with a twist to bring one elbow towards the opposite knee, slowly lower yourself back to the floor, repeat in the other direction, then relax.

Precautions
As for the previous exercises. Take care to start the twisting movement as soon as you lift your head and shoulders off the ground.

Effects
This movement strengthens the oblique abdominal and trunk muscles on either side of your body. Concentric strength is improved as you lift the weight of your trunk, head and arms against gravity, eccentric strength as you control the reverse movement. These muscles are specially important if you do activities involving twisting, such as racket sports, games which involve kicking, or throwing events.

As a test
1 Can you perform the movement properly, without pain? Is it easier going in one direction than in the other?
2 If the movement is painless, count the number of repetitions you can do over one minute.

As an exercise
Start with ten repetitions (i.e. five to either side); build up to five sets of ten repetitions.

5. Hip extension lying on your back with knees bent (crook-lying, or hook-lying)

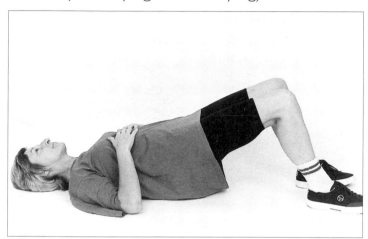

Lie on your back with your knees bent, feet flat on the floor and hands resting across your midriff – this position is technically called 'crook-lying'. Lift your hips off the floor with control, then slowly lower and relax completely.

Precautions
Do not lift your hips too high or arch your back hard. Stop if you feel any pain at all.

Effects
The back extensor, gluteal and hamstring muscles are strengthened together with the lower part of the shoulder girdle. The muscle work is concentric as you lift the weight of your pelvis up against gravity, eccentric as you control the reverse movement.

As a test
1 Can you do the movement properly without pain?
2 If you can, count the number of repetitions you can achieve over one minute.

As an exercise
Start with ten repetitions, build up to three sets of fifteen repetitions.

6. Hip extension lying with one knee bent, one leg straight (half-crook-lying)

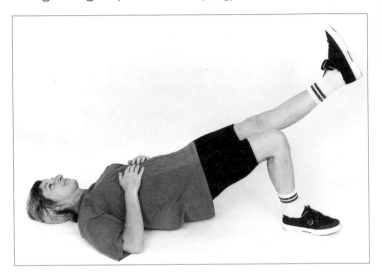

Lie on your back with one leg straight, the other bent with the foot flat on the floor: this position is technically termed 'half-crook-lying'. Lift your hips and the straight leg off the supporting surface, slowly lower, and relax completely. Repeat, reversing the position of the legs.

Precautions
Keep your hips and knees level. Do not arch your back, but stop when your abdomen is in line with your thighs. Stop immediately if there is any pain.

Effects
This is a co-ordination exercise which strengthens the back extensors and hip extensors (gluteal and hamstring muscles) on one side as they support the weight of your pelvis and trunk up to the lower shoulder girdle, while the unsupported side holds the balance using the hip and knee muscles to hold the straight leg up against gravity. The back extensors, gluteals and hamstrings on the weightbearing, supported side work concentrically as you lift your hips against gravity, and eccentrically as you control the reverse movement. On the unsupported side, where the leg is straight, the hip flexors, knee extensors and ankle dorsiflexors (on top of the leg and hip) work isometrically (statically) to hold the leg up against gravity.

As a test

1 Can you do the movement properly and without pain? Is it easier to do on one side than the other?
2 If it is painless, count the number of repetitions you can do over one minute, first on one side, then the other.

As an exercise
Start with five repetitions each way, and build up to three sets of fifteen repetitions.

7. Hip extension with abdomen supported

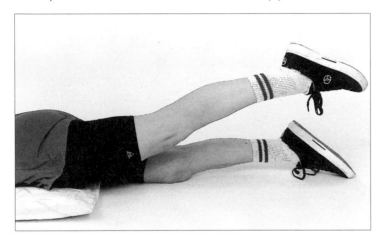

Lying on your stomach with a pillow under your hips and abdomen, lift one leg a little way up behind you, keeping the knee locked straight and pointing your toes to extend your foot; slowly lower, relax. Repeat with the other leg.

Precautions
Do not try to lift your legs to the highest limit, especially if your lower back is very flexible and can arch backwards to a great degree. Restrict the movement to a very small range, even if you feel you can lift further. Do not work through pain.

Effects
This strengthens the hamstring and gluteal muscles concentrically through a small range of movement as they lift the weight of your leg against gravity, and eccentrically as you reverse the movement with control. The back extensors are activated to stabilize the back while the leg moves at the hip joint. It is also a co-ordination exercise for the hip and knee:

if you have had knee problems, you may find it difficult to keep the knee locked straight, so you have to concentrate on this element of the movement.

As a test
1 Can you perform the movement properly on each side, without pain? Is it more difficult on one side than the other?
2 If you can do the movement without pain, count the repetitions you can achieve in one minute.

As an exercise
Start with ten repetitions on one side, then the other; build up to three sets of fifteen repetitions. Progress by adding light weights, either on your feet or strapped to your ankles, and then increase the weights in easy stages.

8. Hip extension lying flat on your stomach (prone-lying)

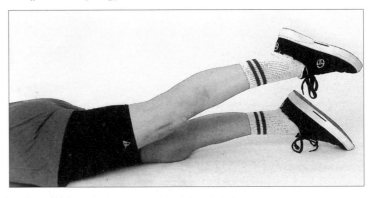

Lying on your stomach, lift one leg up behind you with the knee locked straight, toes pointed and foot extended in line with your body; slowly lower the leg, then relax completely. Repeat with the other leg.

Precautions
Do not try to lift more than a little way, even if you think you can. You must not feel that you have stretched to the limit of your available joint movement. The movement has to be very small range indeed. Do not work through pain.

Effects
This exercise is an advanced version of the preceding one, and is usually harder to do, if you have had a back problem. It strengthens the hamstring and gluteal muscles concentri-

cally in a very small movement (not more than 15 degrees) as you lift the weight of your leg against gravity, and eccentrically as you slowly put the leg down. Technically, the movement takes place in the muscles' *inner range*. It improves muscle tone in the hip and back extensor muscles, and so helps the stability of the lower back joints.

As a test
1 Can you perform the movement accurately without pain, and equally on both sides?
2 If you can, count your repetitions over one minute.

As an exercise
Start with ten repetitions, lifting each leg alternately, and build up to three sets of twenty repetitions. Progress by using light weights on your feet or strapped to your ankles, and gradually increase the weights in easy stages.

9. Trunk extension with abdomen supported

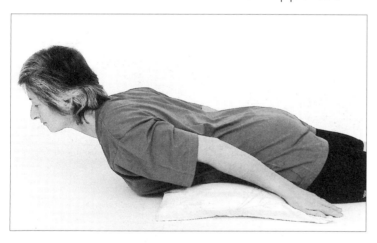

Lying on your stomach with a pillow under your hips and abdomen, and your arms relaxed alongside you, palms down facing the floor, lift your head and shoulders a little way upwards (backwards); gently press your shoulder blades together, keeping your hands in contact with the supporting surface; slowly lower, relax.

Precautions
Do not lift your trunk more than a little way, even if you feel you could lift further. As you bring the shoulder blades together, make sure that you do not strain or lift your head

and shoulders higher off the ground. Keep your elbows straight, and your hands relaxed throughout the movement. Your palms can face down on to the supporting surface, or you can have them facing upwards, or in neutral alongside your body according to which position you find more natural or comfortable. Do not work through pain.

Effects

This strengthens your back extensor muscles from the lower back up to the shoulder girdle, neck and head concentrically as you lift the weight of your trunk against gravity, and eccentrically on the controlled reverse. This improves the muscle tone and enhances the joint stability.

As a test

1 Can you achieve the movement accurately and without pain?
2 If you can, count the repetitions you can achieve over one minute.

As an exercise

Start with ten repetitions, and build up to three sets of twenty.

10. Trunk extension flat on your stomach (prone-lying)

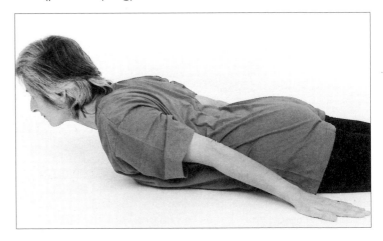

Lying flat on your stomach, with your arms relaxed alongside you, palms flat on the ground, lift your head and shoulders just a little way upwards, bring the shoulder blades together; slowly lower, and relax.

Precautions

Be very careful not to lift too high or arch your back forcibly. The movement should feel perfectly comfortable and well within the limits of your natural joint range capacity. Do not work through pain.

Effects

This movement strengthens the back extensor and shoulder girdle muscles concentrically in a very small, inner range as you lift the weight of your trunk, shoulders and head against gravity, and eccentrically as you lower your trunk with control. It promotes stability in all the spinal joints, and helps to counteract the normal compressive effect of gravity acting downwards on to the spinal column. It is especially important for establishing the right muscle balance between the shoulder blades, ribs and spine.

As a test

1 Can you do the movement accurately and without pain?
2 If you can, count the number of repetitions you can achieve over one minute.

As an exercise

Start with ten repetitions, and build up to three sets of twenty.

11. Hip abduction in side-lying

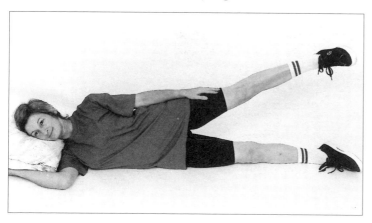

Lying on one side, with your body and legs in a straight line, lift your upper leg upwards (sideways from the body) with the knee locked straight; slowly lower and relax. Repeat with the other leg, lying on the other side.

Precautions

Take care to keep the knee locked and your hip well forward. Your leg should remain in line with your body, so that your hip does not bend and your foot does not come forwards. Do not try to lift the leg too high. Do not work through pain.

Effects

This movement strengthens the hip abductor muscles at the side of the pelvis. The muscle work is concentric as you lift the weight of your leg against gravity, and eccentric as you lower the leg with control in the direction of gravity.

As a test

1 Can you do the movement correctly, without pain, and equally on either side?
2 If you can, count the number of repetitions you can achieve in one minute, first on one side, then the other.

As an exercise

Start with ten repetitions on one side, then the other. Build up to three sets of twenty repetitions on each side. To progress, use a light weight on your foot or strapped to your ankle, and increase the weight in gradual stages.

12. The side-raise

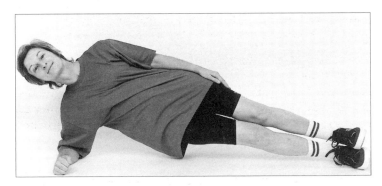

Lying on one side, resting on your elbow, lift your hips up sideways so that you are balanced on your elbow and the side of your foot; slowly lower your hips, then relax. Repeat on the other side.

Precautions

Do not try to lift your hips too high. As you lift your hips take care to keep your body in line. Do not try this if you have any shoulder problems. Do not work through pain.

Effects

This movement strengthens the side of your body which is closest to the floor, as you lift the weight of your trunk and legs against gravity. It works especially the hip abductors, trunk side flexors and latissimus dorsi. These muscles are strengthened concentrically as you lift your hips and eccentrically as you reverse the movement with control. The exercise is important for establishing a good balance on either side of your pelvis and trunk.

As a test

1 Can you do the movement correctly without pain? Can you achieve the same range of movement equally easily on both sides?
2 If you can perform the movement without pain, count the number of repetitions you can do in one minute on one side, then the other.

As an exercise

Start with five repetitions on one side, then the other. Build up to three sets of ten repetitions on each side.

13. Standing hip abduction

Standing on one leg, lift the other leg sideways a short distance, keeping the knee straight, slowly lower the leg without putting the foot to the floor, then repeat the sideways movement six times, with control. Repeat standing on the other leg.

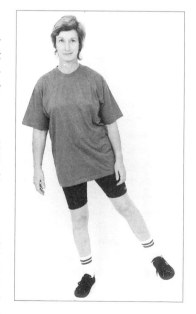

Precautions

Stand close to a wall or support, at the side you are balancing on, in case you overbalance. Keep your body straight and your moving leg in line sideways with your body. Do not work through pain.

Effects

The hip abductor muscles at the side of the hip and pelvis on the moving leg work concentrically as you lift the weight of the leg against gravity, and eccentrically as you lower the leg with control. The same muscles on the supporting side work isometrically to hold your pelvis horizontally in line while the other leg moves. All the balance mechanisms in the standing leg from the foot and ankle to the hip and lower back are activated.

The movement requires good balance and co-ordination throughout the body, as well as muscle strength around the pelvis. If your balance is poor on one or both sides, your shock-absorbing mechanisms for sports involving running and jumping may not be able to work as well as they should. If there is an imbalance, compensation by other muscles will cause greater pressure on the hip and lower back during physical activities. This can affect either the weaker or the stronger side, according to the nature of the exercise.

As a test

1 Can you do the movement fluently without pain? Is it more difficult on one side than the other?
2 If you can do the exercise without pain, count the number of repetitions you can achieve in the space of half a minute, first on one leg, then the other.

As an exercise

Start with the six basic movements, and build up to three sets of ten to fifteen movements on each side. To progress, you can strap a light weight on to the ankle of the moving leg, and later increase the weight in gradual stages.

14. Shoulder abduction

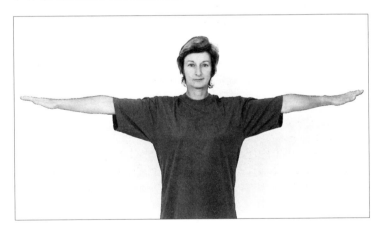

Sitting or standing with your arms by your sides, lift both arms straight out sideways to horizontal, keeping your neck muscles relaxed. Slowly lower your arms to your sides, then relax completely.

Precautions

Take care not to let your neck muscles (trapezii) tense up. You may need to watch yourself in a mirror to prevent this. If you find it difficult to lift your arms without contracting the neck muscles, try bending your elbows and lifting just a little way, then gradually build up to doing the full movement as you get the feeling of how to do it. Do not work through pain.

Effects

This movement strengthens your shoulder abductor muscles (the deltoid and supraspinatus muscles on each side). They work concentrically as you raise your arms, and eccentrically as you lower them with control. Relaxing the neck muscles is especially important because it establishes the correct relationship between the neck and shoulder muscles. All too often, the correct pattern of movement in these muscles is distorted, and the neck muscles are activated when the shoulder muscles should be working. This happens if you have to work with your hands while keeping your arms close to your sides or forwards from your body, for instance while typing, sewing or operating a checkout till. It can also happen through tension, as your neck muscles then tighten and come into play as soon as you try to use your arms, reversing the correct pattern which should allow your arm muscles to be activated first. Overactive neck muscles can be associated with, or contribute to neck pain.

As a test

1 Can you perform the movement accurately, without pain?
2 If you can, how many repetitions can you achieve in the space of one minute?

As an exercise

Start with five repetitions, and gradually build up to three sets of ten. When you are confident that you can do the movement perfectly, without tensing the neck muscles, you can use light weights, either held in your hands or strapped to your wrists.

15. Shoulder mobility

Sitting or standing, lift one arm above your head, bend your elbow and place your hand, palm down towards your body, behind your upper back; keeping your other arm close to your side, place that (second) hand behind your back, palm up, and bend your elbow to bring your hands together or close to each other. Hold the position for a count of three, then repeat in the opposite direction.

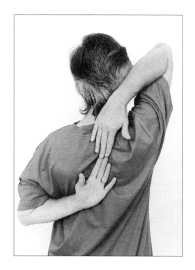

Precautions

Try to keep your head up and straight. Do not force the movement. Do not work through pain.

Effects

This movement stretches and twists your shoulders. The dominant arm is usually slightly limited compared to the non-dominant, especially in people who have consistently used their arm forcibly, such as racket games players and throwers (discus and javelin throwers, baseball pitchers, cricket bowlers). With age, this shoulder stiffness tends to get worse, unless remedial exercises are done. The exercises are necessary, because shoulder limitation can cause more strain through the upper or lower back, or both, when full arm movements are attempted.

As a test

1 Can you do the movement on either side without pain?
2 Do your hands overlap, or is there a gap between the fingers of each hand?

As an exercise

Stretch your hands behind your back and hold the position for a count of six. Repeat ten times on each side. If the exercise is more difficult in one direction than the other, do six repetitions in the more difficult position, to three the other way, and gradually build up to twenty movements (difficult side) as against ten (easy side).

16. Sitting hip adductor stretch

Sitting on a mat on the floor, place the soles of your feet together and bring your heels towards your body, keeping your back straight, head up; with your hands over your feet, elbows resting on your thighs, let your knees relax gently sideways as far as they comfortably can.

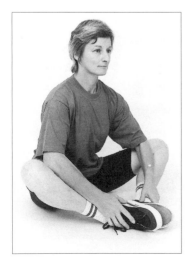

Precautions

Do not force any part of this movement. Do not work through pain.

Effects

This exercise stretches the adductor muscles on the inner thighs. If these muscles are tight, they limit your range of hip movement. If one side is tighter than the other, the hip on that side will be relatively limited, creating muscle imbalance affecting the pelvis and lower back. Hip injuries or conditions such as osteoarthritis can cause spasm and tightness in the adductor muscles. A tear or direct injury to the muscles themselves can also result in shortening. Good flexibility in the adductors is necessary to allow the hips full and symmetrical function.

As a test
Marks are made on the floor to show the position of your seat and heels. The vertical distance from your knees to the floor is measured on either side. When you get up, the distance between the markers is measured and recorded, so that you sit in the same position for the re-test.

As an exercise
Hold the stretched position absolutely still for a count of six. Repeat at least five times, or ten times if your adductors are especially tight.

17. Sit-and-reach stretch

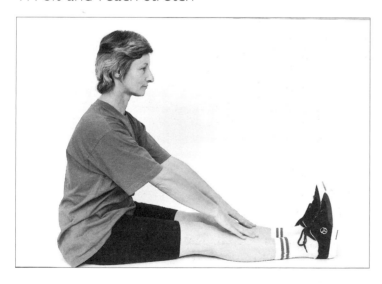

Sitting on the floor with your legs straight in front of you (technically this position is called 'long-sitting'), reach forwards to slide your hands down your legs, keeping your arms and back straight, your head up. Hold the position for a count of six, then relax completely.

Precautions
Do not attempt the movement if you have pain simply sitting with your legs straight. Do not force the movement, or try to

reach your toes if you have to bend your back and curve your shoulders to do so. Do not try to push further into the stretch from the already stretched position.

Effects

This movement, done properly, stretches your hamstring muscles. If your hamstrings are very long and flexible, you may be able to reach beyond your toes. If they are short and tight, you may have difficulty in sitting up with your legs at right angles to your body. Tight hamstrings exert a drag on your pelvis through your seat-bones (ischial tuberosities), pulling the pelvis into a backward tilt. Stretching the hamstrings is vital to counteract this. If you cannot achieve the movement at all, you have to use those of the alternative hamstring stretches which you can do without discomfort (see pp.194–5).

As a test

1 Can you get into position and reach forwards to some degree without pain?
2 If you can, the distance from your middle finger to your big toe on either side is measured.

As an exercise

Repeat the stretch five times at first, and build up gradually to three sets of five repetitions.

18. Prone-lying trunk extension stretch

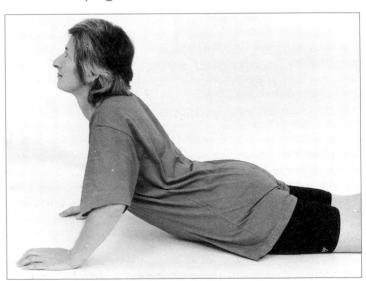

Lying on your stomach, place your hands under your shoulders, palms down on the floor; resting on your hands, gently lift your shoulders and upper trunk upwards as far as you can, keeping your hips on the floor and your head up. Hold for a count of six, then relax completely.

Precautions
Do not attempt this movement if you have pain lying flat on your stomach. Do not force the movement or arch your back hard. Do not try to push further into the stretch from the stretched position.

Effects
This movement stretches the hip flexor and lower abdominal muscles over the front of your hips and trunk. If these muscles are very long and flexible, and your spinal joints very mobile, you may be able to arch your back to a considerable degree. If they are tight and your spinal joints stiff, you may have difficulty lifting your trunk upwards at all. Hip flexor tightness combined with abdominal muscle weakness tends to drag the pelvis into a forward tilt, often creating an excessive curve in the back (lumbar lordosis). Stretching the hips is important for counteracting this.

As a test
1 Can you lie in position on your stomach and lift yourself up to any degree without pain?
2 If you can, the vertical distance between the floor and the top of your breast-bone (sternum) is measured. A second measurement may be made, between the floor and your chin.

As an exercise
Repeat the stretch five times at first, building up gradually to three sets of five repetitions.

19. Prone-lying front thigh stretch

Lying on your stomach, bend one knee and hold your ankle with your hand on the same side; gently pull your heel towards your bottom (buttock), until you feel a *slight* pulling sensation down your front thigh muscles. Hold the stretched position for a count of six, then relax completely. Repeat with the other leg.

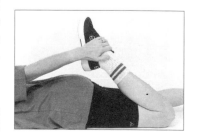

Precautions
Do not attempt this movement if you have pain lying flat on your stomach. Do not pull your foot hard, even if you feel

you could stretch further. If it is difficult, or hurts your back to reach your ankle with your hands, loop a belt around the ankle and pull the ends of the belt gently to achieve the stretch. Do not increase the stretch from the already stretched position.

Effects

This movement stretches the front thigh muscles which cross the knee and the hip. If your thighs are very flexible, you may need to place a small support under the thigh just above the knee to provide greater stretch over the front of the hip. If your front thigh muscles are tight, they interfere with the balance between the knee and the hip, and can contribute to excessive forward tilting of the pelvis, therefore increasing the curvature of the lower back. Stretching the front thigh is therefore important for protecting the knees, hips and pelvis.

As a test

1 Can you lie in position and pull your foot back to bend your knee without pain?
2 If you can, the distance between your heel and the highest point of your seat is measured on either side.

As an exercise

Repeat the stretch five times at first, building up to three sets of five repetitions.

20. Front-shoulder stretch

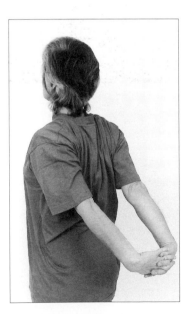

Sitting or standing, place your hands behind your back and clasp your hands together; keeping your elbows straight and your head up, lift your hands up behind you, until you feel a gentle stretch on the fronts of your shoulders. Hold the stretch for a count of six, then relax completely.

Precautions

Do not work through pain. Take care to keep your back straight, head up. Do not force the movement so that your upper back has to bend forwards as you lift your arms.

Effects

This stretches the fronts of your shoulders, which tend to tighten with excessive use, such as intensive tennis playing, or the effects of ageing. If the shoulders are allowed to tighten, they pull the arm-bones slightly forwards. This can cause stress on the upper back (thoracic region) and neck (cervical region) during activities involving full movements of the arms. Therefore it is important to maintain flexibility in the fronts of the shoulders.

As a test

1 Can you take up the position and lift your arms behind you without discomfort?
2 If you can, the distance between your outermost third knuckle and the most prominent part of your seat (buttock) is measured.

As an exercise

Repeat the stretch five times at first, building up gradually to three sets of five repetitions.

21. Hanging

Place your hands over a hanging bar, with palms facing downwards; holding the bar with your hands to take your weight, relax your body and let your trunk stretch. Hold the position for a few seconds, or until your arms start to feel tired, then step down.

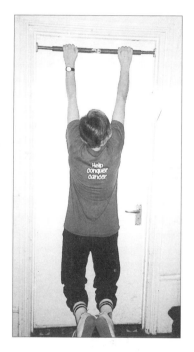

Precautions

Do not attempt this exercise if it causes pain. Do not try it if you have had recent neck problems. If you use a bar which is set high off the floor so that you can hang with your legs straight under you, do not jump down at the end of the exercise, but make sure that you can step down on to a support and then to the floor. If you have a low bar (for instance set in a doorway), bend your knees behind you to take your feet off the floor, but try not to arch your back too much, or to the point of discomfort.

Effects

Hanging by the arms allows the spinal joints, especially in the lower back, to stretch downwards under the effect of gravity. This has the effect of decompressing the joints, by reversing the usual compressive influence of gravity. It can be very useful for relieving stiffness in the spinal joints.

As a test

1 Can you get into position and take your bodyweight through your hands without discomfort?
2 If you can, time how long you can maintain a relaxed hanging position.

As an exercise

Repeat the hanging stretch just a few (say three to five) times to start with. Gradually increase the amount of time you spend hanging for each repetition as your arms get stronger.

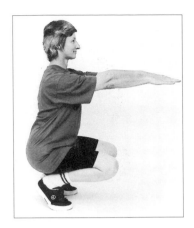

22. Standing squats

Standing straight, with your feet parallel and slightly apart, go up on your toes, and staying on your toes, bend your knees with control to squat down as fully as you can, then straighten your knees quickly to stand up again; finally, let your heels down to the floor and relax completely.

Precautions

Keep your back as straight as you can during the movement. If your balance is poor, stand close to a support. Make sure your knees bend symmetrically: if one is stiffer than the other, stop the movement when the limit of the stiffer joint is reached. Straighten your knees hard to lock your knee-caps at the end of the movement, and then relax them, to avoid knee-cap pain. Do not do the movement if it causes any pain in your legs or back.

Effects

This movement strengthens your front thigh muscles, especially the quadriceps group, and the seat muscles (gluteals). They work eccentrically as you control the knee-bending movement to lower your bodyweight in the direction of gravity, and concentrically as you straighten your legs to lift your bodyweight against gravity.

The ability to perform this movement is vital for protecting the back. If your legs are weak and you cannot bend your knees easily, it is difficult to lift any object or load from the floor safely, as you will have to bend your back and use the back muscles at a disadvantage. Any activities which involve reaching down to the floor will also make you bend your back in a potentially harmful way. Movement limitation in one or both knee joints also affects your legs' shock-absorbing capacities during walking, running and jumping, so more jarring forces may be transmitted upwards to your hip(s) or lower back. If one knee is not working properly, you may have a limp, which in turn may disrupt the muscle balance of your pelvis and lower back.

As a test

1 Can you do the movement properly without pain?
2 If you can, count the number of full movements you can achieve over one minute.

As an exercise

Start with five repetitions, and build up to three sets of fifteen repetitions. To progress, hold light weights in your hands, by your sides at first, then held straight out in front of you.

Remedial exercises for the back, neck and related joints

9

REASONS FOR DOING REMEDIAL EXERCISES

Remedial exercises restore normal or better movement to parts which have been undermined by pain, damage or both. The human body is an active machine, depending on muscle actions and joint movements in order to function efficiently. Pain or injury which affects bone, joint, muscle or any tissue in the spine can result in an increase in muscle tone in the affected area, causing muscle tightness or spasm. A drop in muscle tone can occur instead of muscle spasm, or in many cases muscle weakness or low tone follows once the spasm has gone.

Throughout the body, you need to balance joint mobility with a suitable degree of stability. Joint stiffness (hypomobility) can in itself create problems in the structure of the joint, if it is allowed to develop. It has to be controlled through gentle mobilizing exercises, at the very least to prevent the stiffness from getting worse. Hypermobile joints can also become problematical and cause pain, so the excessive range of movement should be limited by exercises designed to create better joint stability.

An active rehabilitation programme is essential for full recovery from injury, or after surgery for a physical problem. It is also vital in certain medical conditions. Ankylosing spondylitis (see p.146), for instance, is an arthritic condition for which the only effective treatment is a comprehensive programme of protective exercises to maintain good joint range, muscle strength and flexibility, and overall body balance. In fact, all back and neck sufferers should cultivate the habit of daily exercise which is the discipline required to control not only ankylosing spondylitis, but also many other types of spinal pain.

Remedial exercises are also valuable because they provide a daily reminder that you need to be aware of looking after yourself in relation to your current or previous problem. Having to focus on your exercise programme every day can serve to motivate you to maintain good postural habits.

> Pain means
> no gain

WHEN NOT TO DO REMEDIAL EXERCISES

Although full recovery from a spinal problem depends on an accurate remedial and protective programme of exercises, there are certain situations in which exercises of any kind are inappropriate and should not be done. In the active inflammatory stages of some arthritic conditions such as rheumatoid arthritis, the joints become very tender and oversensitive, and exercise or movement only exacerbates the pain in the inflamed joints. In mechanical problems involving nerve root disturbance with referred pain into the arm(s) or leg(s), exercises can also make the pain much worse. Exercises are also contra-indicated if you are ill, suffering from any kind of infection which requires antibiotic treatment, or feeling exceptionally tired and run-down.

WHEN AND HOW TO DO REMEDIAL EXERCISES

A systematic regime is essential for achieving the aims of any rehabilitation exercise programme. You should try to discipline yourself to do a regular sequence of exercises, preferably twice or three times a day. At the very least, some of the remedial exercises you have been set should be done every day without fail.

Remedial exercises should *never* cause pain. If you are recommended to do exercises and find that they are painful, you should modify them, in case you are doing them incorrectly. If they still cause pain, stop and report back to your practitioner as quickly as possible. Sometimes active sports players try too hard and force the therapeutic exercise movements, on the assumption that exercises have to hurt to do you good. This is mistaken. On the contrary, you should feel little immediate effect when you do remedial exercises. You are safest if you feel you have not done enough.

A remedial exercise programme should be progressive. Start with just a few repetitions of each exercise that you are recommended to do, and then build up the repetitions and sets as you become familiar with the movements. Every movement has to be accurate. If you are short of time, cut down the number of exercises you set yourself to do, rather than trying to cram them all in too quickly.

Remedial exercises must be done in a positive frame of mind. You will be better motivated if you constantly remind yourself that the programme is making you better and will help protect you from future back or neck problems. Thinking positively also helps the flow of blood through the injured area, which can be a significant factor in functional recovery. Concentration is important, to ensure that you perform every part of every exercise absolutely correctly, as quality of movement is essential in remedial exercises.

Besides doing the exercises as a special daily routine, it is also useful to incorporate certain of the movements into any overall exercise or training programme you normally do. Many of the exercises are suitable for warming-up and warming-down, others could be added into aerobic or weight-training schedules. The hanging exercises are especially useful for counteracting the compressive effects of heavy weight training, rugby tackling or rowing, for instance. The stretching exercises are useful if you have a tendency to be inflexible, or if your sport does not provide a wide range of movements. The remedial exercises are also protective, so they should be maintained for as long as possible even after you have recovered from a specific back or neck problem. The most important time to do protective exercises is after any strenuous sports or training sessions.

Warning

- Always be guided by your practitioner as to which exercises to do, how many, and how often
- Never persevere with exercises which cause or increase pain either in your back or neck, or anywhere else in your body

DANGEROUS EXERCISES

It is a mistake to be dogmatic about which exercises might be safe or dangerous for the spinal joints. Opinions differ, and there are no hard and fast rules beyond the hints given by experience and common sense.

My personal views on exercises I consider 'dangerous' or potentially harmful for the back and neck are guided by objective principles relating to biomechanics, and clinical experience of exercises which have caused or aggravated spinal problems in patients. If you have been recommended to do exercises that are listed here as possibly dangerous, check with your practitioner that they are indeed safe for you. If in doubt, be guided by the practitioner treating you, or seek a further opinion from another practitioner, preferably through your doctor.

The double-leg-raise done lying on your back is problematical for two reasons: first, as you lift the legs from the floor, the hip flexors tighten and force the low back to arch, causing a big increase in pressure in the joints; second, there is also a large increase in the pressure inside your abdomen because the abdominal muscles have to work very strongly isometrically to hold the position once your legs are lifted. The exercise carries the risks of causing injury to the low back, or a hernia through the abdominal wall or in the groin. These risks are present even of you have been doing this exercise routinely for a long time, as it is not a protective movement.

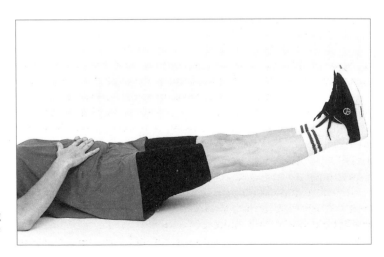

Lifting both legs upwards while lying down places excessive strain on the back and abdomen

Lying on your back, keeping your hips on the floor and doing cycling movements with your legs in the air does not seem to carry the same injury risks as double-leg-raising, but if you do the cycling movements balanced on your shoulders and head, so that your trunk is vertical, there is dangerous compression on the top of your upper back and on your neck. This is also true of the exercise in which you lie on your back and take your legs right over your head so that your toes touch the floor behind your head. You have to be very experienced at doing this movement, which should only ever be done on a well-cushioned mat, to avoid the risk of injuring your upper back.

Lying on your stomach and forcing your body upwards into extension can cause dangerous compression in the spinal joints, and this can damage the discs or other joint structures. The problem is partly the excessive range of movement which forces the spinal joints into extreme ranges, and partly the muscle effort involved.

When you do spinal exercises standing up, gravity plays a significant part in compressing the joints vertically. Any forcible movements in any direction can cause over-strain in the spinal joints, damaging the joint structures. As forward bending allows the greatest range of movement for the spine, it is in this position that most harm can be done, although it is also possible to cause injury through harsh side-bending and backward-bending movements as well. The compression effects are of course magnified if you do the exercises with weights in your hands or on your shoulders.

Pool exercises

Swimming is an excellent form of exercise for the recovery stages following a back or neck problem. If you enjoy swimming, it can also help psychologically. However, you should not create tension by trying to do serious training, swimming lengths at full pelt using only one stroke. It is best to swim in a relaxed way, trying to use as many strokes as possible, to create a wide variety of movements and to avoid repetitive patterns which might cause stress on the spine.

It is also possible and helpful to do exercises in the pool, apart from swimming. You can do movement patterns for the whole body, and quite often it is possible to do certain exercises in the pool before you can achieve them without pain on land. Even people who do not know how to swim can safely stand in a hydrotherapy (rehabilitation) pool or the shallow end of a swimming pool using floats or a buoyancy jacket in order to do movements in the water. The effects of exercising in water are quite complex. The buoyancy of the water provides support, and therefore assists your movements if you do them slowly close to the surface of the water. If you make quick movements you create turbulence which provides resistance. When you perform movements below the surface, the resistance provided by the water increases with depth.

As hydrotherapy is quite specialized, it is best to do pool exercises under the guidance of a qualified practitioner, usually a chartered physiotherapist (physical therapist). Using buoyancy aids, even if you are a good swimmer, you can isolate parts of the body in order to exercise them. For instance, with your upper body and neck well supported, you can do low back, hip and leg movements floating on the surface of the water, facing upwards or downwards. Using floats to support the legs and trunk, you can do exercises for the arms, shoulder region, neck and head. Floating on the surface of the water, you can do movements on the surface or into the water from the surface. Holding the rail and standing up in the water, you can do a wide variety of movements involving any of the body's joints, using the effects of increased resistance provided by the depth of the water.

Very often, you will feel relaxed after a good pool session, and joints in your back and neck which felt stiff beforehand will feel much freer. However, you have to be careful, as the freedom of movement you gain in the pool can lead to a bad reaction of pain shortly after the session. If you experience this, you have done too much in a session. To avoid the backlash, you should try to end each pool session with the feeling that you could have done more. You have to be especially careful not to do too many mobilizing exercises, even though it is tempting to explore the enjoyable feeling of joint freedom that the water creates. You should rest lying down for up to an hour after remedial pool exercises.

In most cases you should not do pool sessions on consecutive days, although daily sessions may be prescribed for certain conditions.

EARLY-STAGE STRENGTHENING AND MOBILIZING EXERCISES

1 Lie on your back with your knees bent, gently flatten your back so that your whole spine is in contact with the mat, then arch your back to lift it slightly off the floor. Repeat 5–20 times.
Strengthens the low back extensor and the abdominal muscles, while gently mobilizing the low back)

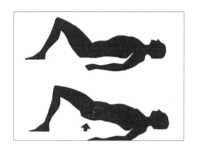

2 Lie on your back with your knees bent, lift your hips upwards off the mat a little way, then slowly lower them back. Repeat 5–20 times. *(Strengthens the low back, gluteal and hamstring muscles)*

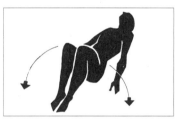

3 Lie on your back with your knees bent and close together, gently roll your knees over to one side, then bring them back to roll the other way. Repeat 5–20 times. *(Mobilizes the low back)*

4 Lie on your back with your knees bent and slightly apart, stretch your arms forwards towards your knees and lift your trunk gently upwards to slide your hands closer to your knees, keeping your head in line with your trunk, then slowly lower your upper body back again. Repeat 5–20 times. *(Strengthens the abdominal muscles and co-ordinates the abdominals with the gluteals and hamstrings)*

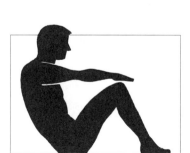

5 Lie on your back with your knees bent and close together, lift your knees a little way up so that your feet just leave the floor, then slowly lower them down again, keeping your knees bent throughout the movement. Repeat 5–20 times. *(Strengthens the lower abdominal muscles)*

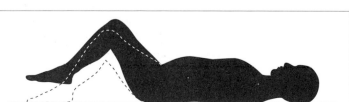

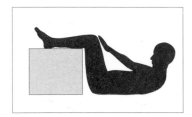

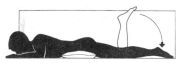

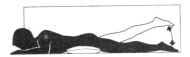

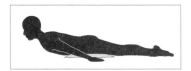

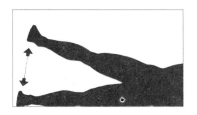

6 Lie on your back with your knees bent to right angles and supported up on a chair or stool. Lift your head and shoulders just a little, and stretch your hands towards your knees, then slowly lower back to the starting position. Repeat 5–20 times.
(Strengthens your front neck and upper abdominal muscles)

7 Lie on your stomach with a pillow under your hips, bend one knee, slowly straighten the leg again, then repeat with the other leg. Repeat 10–20 times.
(Strengthens the hamstrings and activates the extensor muscles in the low back isometrically)

8 Lie on your stomach with a pillow under your hips, lift one leg up backwards a very short way, keeping the knee locked straight, slowly lower the leg back, then repeat with the other leg. Repeat 5–20 times.
(Strengthens the hamstring, gluteal and extensor muscles on each side)

9 Lie on your stomach with a pillow under your hips, lift your head and shoulders a little way backwards, keeping your head in line with your upper back and your hands on the supporting surface, press your shoulder blades gently together, then slowly lower your trunk down again. Repeat 5–20 times.
(Strengthens the back extensor, neck and shoulder girdle muscles)

10 Lie on one side with your head on a pillow and another pillow between your knees; keeping your knee locked straight and your hips well forward, lift your upper leg a little way, then slowly lower it down again. Repeat 5–20 times on one side, then the other.
(Strengthens the hip abductor muscles on the uppermost leg)

11 Kneeling on all fours, gently arch your back so that it forms a hump upwards and tuck your head down towards your chest; then lift your head as you let your back curve gently downwards. Repeat 10–20 times.

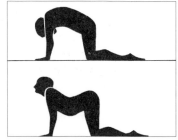

(Strengthens the back extensor and abdominal muscles while gently mobilizing the whole spine from pelvis to neck)

12 Kneeling on all fours, stretch one leg out sideways with the toe touching the floor, and turn your head towards that leg so that you can see the foot over your shoulder; swing the foot gently round in an arc behind you, keeping your knee straight and your toe close to the floor, and turn your head at the same time to the other side; repeat the movement three times with one leg, then change your position to repeat the cycle with your other leg. Repeat 6–10 times in all.

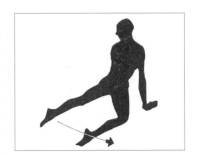

(Gently mobilizes the hip, sacroiliac region and side of the trunk)

13 Sitting or standing, keeping your back straight, gently tuck your chin down on to your chest, then straighten your head up and tip it slightly backwards so that you look up. Repeat 5–10 times.

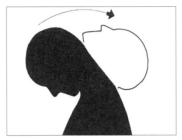

(Strengthens the neck muscles and gently mobilizes the neck joints in the forward-backward direction)

14 Sitting or standing, with your back straight, tuck your chin down towards your chest and gently turn your head from side to side, keeping your chin down. Repeat 5–10 times.

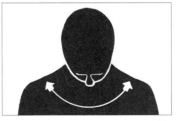

(Strengthens and stretches the neck muscles, especially the rotators)

15 Standing up straight, slowly bend your knees to the half-squatting position, then quickly straighten up again, keeping your back straight.
Repeat 5–20 times.
(Strengthens your quadriceps and gluteal muscles)

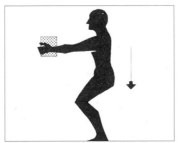

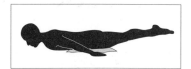

INTERMEDIATE-STAGE STRENGTHENING AND MOBILIZING EXERCISES

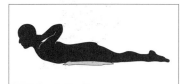

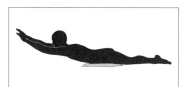

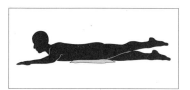

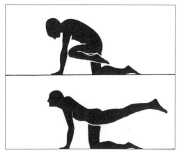

1 Lying on your stomach with a pillow under your hips, lift both legs up backwards just a little way, keeping your knees locked straight, then slowly lower them down. Repeat 5–20 times. Add in light weights strapped to your ankles when the exercise becomes easy.
(Strengthens your hamstring, gluteal and back extensor muscles)

2 Lying on your stomach with a pillow under your hips, place your hands lightly behind your neck and lift your arms, head and upper trunk upwards a little way; lift your elbows to press your shoulder blades together slightly, then slowly lower down. Repeat 5–20 times.
(Strengthens your upper back, neck and shoulder girdle muscles)

3 Lying on your stomach with a pillow under your hips, stretch your arms straight forwards above your head, in line with your trunk, and lift your arms, head and upper body a little way upwards, then slowly lower your body down again. Repeat 5–20 times.
(Strengthens your back extensor and shoulder girdle muscles)

4 Lying on your stomach with a pillow under your hips, lift one leg up a little way from the hip, keeping the knee locked straight, slowly take the leg out sideways, back to centre, then slowly lower and relax completely. Repeat 5–20 times, first on one leg, then the other. Add in light weights strapped to your ankles when the exercise becomes easy.
(Strengthens the gluteal muscles, including the hip abductors)

5 Kneeling on all fours, bring one knee forwards and bend your head down so that your forehead approaches the knee, then stretch your leg back straightening your knee out at the same time as you lift your head up. Repeat three times on one side, then change position to do the movement with the other leg. Do this 5–10 times in all.
(Strengthens the extensor, gluteal and hamstring muscles as well as mobilizing the whole spine)

6 Kneeling on all fours, stretch one arm straight forwards away from your head, and the opposite leg straight backwards; hold the arm and leg in line with your trunk for a count of two, then return to the starting position. Repeat with the opposite arm and leg. Do this 5–20 times.
(Strengthens the extensor muscles through the whole spine, and improves balance and co-ordination)

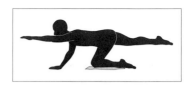

7 Sitting or standing, place the palms of your hands against your forehead, with one hand on top of the other; gently press your hands against your head and tense your neck muscles so that your head does not move. Hold for a count of two, then relax completely. Then place your hands behind your head and press for a count of two, tensing your neck muscles to keep your head still, then relax completely. Repeat 3–6 times.
(Strengthens the front and back neck muscles isometrically for stability)

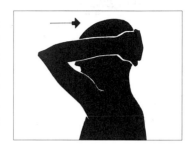

8 Sitting or standing, place your right hand against the right side of your head, covering your ear; gently press your hand against your head, and tense the neck muscles so that your head does not move; hold for a count of two, then relax completely. Next place your left hand against the left side of your head, press gently and tense the neck muscles to resist any movement for a count of two, then relax completely. Repeat 3–6 times.
(Strengthens the side muscles of the neck isometrically for stability)

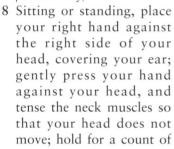

9 Lying on your back on a bench (or bed), with your knees bent and your arms out sideways at right angles to your body, lift your arms vertically upwards to bring your hands together, keeping your elbows straight, then slowly lower outwards again. Repeat 5–20 times, and add in light weights held in your hands when the exercise feels easy.
(Strengthens your chest and front shoulder muscles)

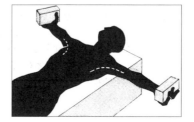

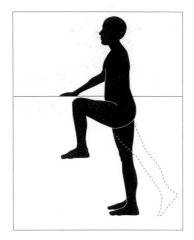

10 Standing with your legs slightly apart and your right hand resting lightly on a bar beside you, bend your left knee and bring the left leg up in front of you towards your chest, then straighten the knee as you take the leg downwards and slightly behind you. Keep your head up and your back as straight as you can. Repeat 5–10 times on one side, then turn round to do the movement on the other side. Add in a light weight strapped to your ankle when the exercise becomes easy.
(Strengthens your leg, hip, gluteal and low back muscles, with hip movement on the moving leg, while the standing side provides stability)

11 Standing with your legs comfortably apart and your hands on your hips, swing your hips round to describe circles, three times to the left, then three times to the right, rhythmically. Repeat 5–20 times.
(Mobilizes the hips and pelvis)

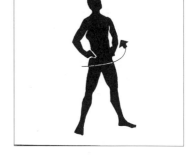

12 Standing with your legs comfortably apart, hold your arms straight out in front of you and turn your upper body to each side in turn in easy continuous movements. Repeat 5–20 times.
(Mobilizes your spine into rotation)

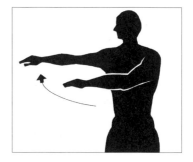

ADVANCED-STAGE STRENGTHENING AND MOBILIZING EXERCISES

Many of these exercises can be used as part of an aerobic training programme if you do enough repetitions sufficiently quickly, but take care to keep the movements accurate.

1 Lying on your stomach with your stomach and legs supported, and your chest and head over the end of the bed or bench, place your hands lightly behind your neck, lower your upper body slowly downwards, then lift up to arch your back slightly, just beyond the horizontal. Use a light weight held in your hands behind your neck when this exercise becomes easy. Repeat 5–15 times.
(Strengthens the back extensor, shoulder girdle and neck muscles through a range of movement)

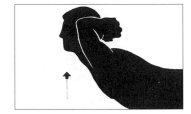

2 Lying on your back with your legs straight and your hands by your sides, bend your knees and lift your legs and head so that they come towards each other, then return with control to the starting position. Repeat 5–20 times.
(Strengthens the abdominal, chest and front neck muscles)

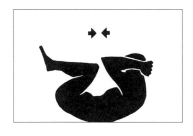

3 Lying on one side, place your elbow under your shoulder with your forearm and hand at right angles to your body; lift your hips upwards, keeping your body straight and your pelvis well forwards, then slowly lower.
Repeat 5–20 times on one side then the other.
(Strengthens the hip abductor and side trunk muscles on the side closest to the ground)

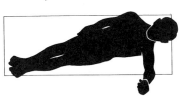

4 Standing, with your elbows bent and kept close to your waist, holding weights in your hands, squat down slowly, then straighten up quickly, keeping your back as straight as you can. Repeat 5–10 times.
(Strengthens your front-thigh muscles while your trunk muscles provide stability)

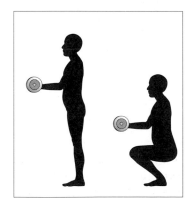

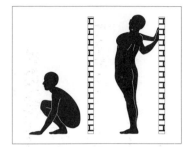

5 Standing about 1 foot (0.3 metre) in front of a wall with your back to it, bend your knees and crouch down to touch the ground with your hands, then stand up again and twist your body to the right to touch the wall behind you with your hands; crouch down again, touch the ground, then straighten and twist to the left to touch the wall with your hands. Repeat 5–20 times.
(Strengthens your legs, and provides co-ordination between your legs, trunk and arms.)

6 Standing with your feet slightly apart and light weights in your hands, bend your knees to crouch down at the same time as you lift your arms forwards and up above your head; straighten up again as you lower your arms, then relax completely. Repeat 5–10 times.

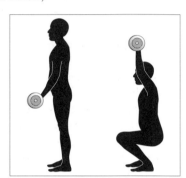

Gradually increase the weights as the exercise becomes easier.
(Strengthens your leg, back and shoulder muscles, using co-ordinated joint movements)

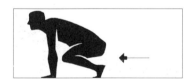

7 Crouch down and place your hands on the ground below your shoulders; balancing on your hands, kick your legs together straight out behind you, then bend your knees to bring them back towards your chest. Repeat the movement 5–20 times before standing up again.
(Strengthens your arms, back and legs, using co-ordinated movements)

8 Lying on your back with your knees slightly bent and your hands resting lightly on either side of your neck, elbows well back, bend your left knee and lift it towards your chest at the same time as you lift your head and shoulders and twist to bring your right elbow towards your left knee; slowly lower back and repeat the movement with the opposite sides. Repeat 5–15 times.
(Strengthens the oblique abdominal and trunk rotator muscles)

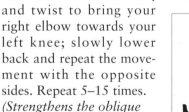
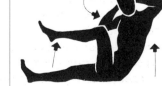

9 Stand in front of a bench about 12 inches (approximately 30 cm) high: the bench can be higher or lower according to your height and fitness level. Holding light weights by your sides in your hands, step up on to the bench with one foot, then the other and straighten your knees, then step down with the first foot, followed by the other, keeping your back as straight as possible throughout. Repeat the movement without stopping 5–20 times leading first with one foot, then the other (10–40 movements in all). Gradually increase the weights as the exercise becomes easy.
(Strengthens your leg and trunk muscles)

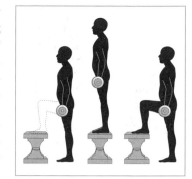

10 Standing up straight with a light weight strapped to one ankle, lift that leg and bend the knee to bring the knee up towards your chest, then straighten the leg and take it behind you, arching your back slightly. Repeat 5–15 times without putting the foot to the floor, then repeat with the other leg. Increase the weight when the exercise becomes easy.
(Strengthens the hip and lower trunk muscles on the moving side, while the other side acts to provide stability)

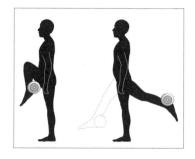

11 Lying on your stomach, place your hands on the ground under your shoulders with your elbows straight, and lift your body off the ground so that you are balanced on your hands and the balls of your feet; slowly bend your elbows, keeping your body straight, to bring your chest towards the ground, then straighten your elbows to lift yourself off the ground again. Repeat 5–15 times.
(Strengthens your trunk and especially the triceps, chest and shoulder girdle muscles)

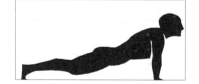

12 Sitting on the ground with your legs straight in front of you, and your upper body leaning backwards, place your hands behind you on the ground, and lift your hips up so that you are balanced on your hands and your heels; bend your elbows to bring your body towards the floor, straighten again, keeping your hips off the floor and repeat 5–15 times before you put your hips down again.
(Strengthens especially the arm, shoulder blade, back extensor and hip extensor muscles)

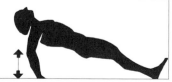
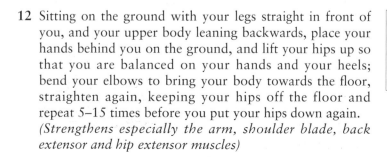

STRETCHING EXERCISES

Stretching exercises should always be done slowly, holding the stretch for about six seconds. Always be guided by the feeling of the muscles at the time. Never push through pain, and never go from the stretched position into a further stretch, as you risk injury. The most you should feel is a slight sensation of gentle pulling over the stretched muscles. You should feel no strain or reaction either during or following a stretch movement. It is especially important to avoid over-stretching the spinal structures.

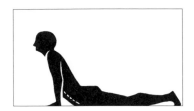

1 Lying on your stomach, place your hands under your shoulders and gently lift your head and shoulders upwards to arch your back as far as is comfortable. Hold for a count of six, relax completely. Repeat 3–6 times.
(Stretches your hip flexor and abdominal muscles)

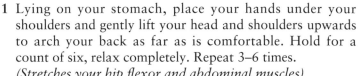

2 Sitting on the floor with your legs apart and the soles of your feet together, place your hands lightly over your ankles, press your knees outwards and lean forwards gently keeping your back straight. Hold for a count of six, relax completely. Repeat 3–6 times.
(Stretches your inner thigh muscles)

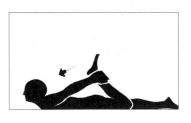

3 Lying on your stomach, bend one knee and hold your ankle with your hand on the same side, or loop a belt round your ankle and hold the ends of the belt; pull your ankle gently towards your bottom, hold for a count of six, then relax completely. Repeat 3–6 times on each leg in turn.
(Stretches the front thigh and hip muscles)

4 Standing on one leg, with your other leg held forwards on a low support, lean gently forwards from the hips, keeping your knees and back straight and your head up, hold for a count of six, then relax completely. Repeat 3–6 times on each leg in turn.
(Stretches the hamstring and gluteal muscles on the forward leg)

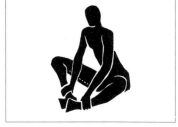

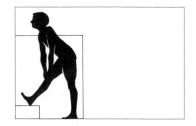

5 Sitting on the floor, bend the right knee and place your right foot on the outside of the left knee, which remains straight out in front of you; with your right arm on the floor beside you, twist your 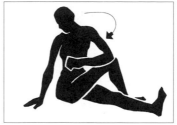 body to the right, and gently press your left elbow against the outside of the bent right knee. Hold for a count of six, then relax completely. Repeat 3–6 times, each side in turn. *(Stretches the hip abductor muscles on the side of the bent knee, and the trunk rotator muscles on the opposite side)*

6 Sitting on a chair or bench, bend forwards from your hips and tuck your head gently down towards your thighs, keeping your hands relaxed by 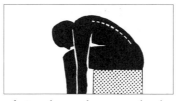 your sides. Hold for a count of six, then relax completely. Repeat 3–6 times. *(Stretches the extensor muscles through the whole spine)*

7 Sitting on the floor with your legs and arms straight in front of you, bend gently forwards from the hips to bring your head down towards your thighs, sliding your hands down towards your feet at the same time. Hold for a count of six, then relax completely. Repeat 3–6 times. *(Stretches the spinal extensor muscles, hamstrings and gluteals)*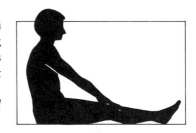

8 Standing, stretch your right arm up above your head and bend your trunk down to the left, sliding your left hand towards your left knee. Hold for a count of six, then relax completely.
Repeat 3–6 times in each direction.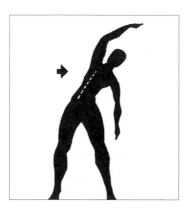
(Stretches the side flexor muscles of the trunk)

9 Lying on your back with both knees bent up towards your chest, place your hands over the tops of your shins, just below your knees, and press your legs gently against your hands for a count of two; relax, releasing your hands from your knees a little, and then pull your knees slowly slightly closer to your body. Repeat 3–6 times.
(Stretches the gluteal and back extensor muscles using a modified hold-relax technique)

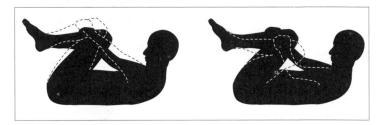

HANGING EXERCISES

Hanging exercises stretch the spine from the shoulders downwards. They are not suitable if you have high blood pressure, weak arms, or neck pain. In some cases they can relieve low back pain, although if they are done in the wrong situation or too soon in a back problem, they can aggravate pain. They can be done using a self-fixing hanging bar, wall-bars or a door-frame provided it is strong enough to take your weight. Your hanging bar may not be high enough for you to stretch out with your legs straight, but the exercises can be done with your knees bent up behind you.

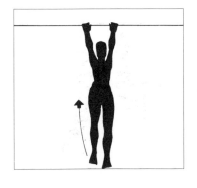

1 Hang by the hands from a bar, keeping your neck as relaxed as possible, and let your trunk relax. Step down as soon as your hands get tired or if you feel tension in your back. Repeat 1–5 times.
(Relaxes the joints in the spine, helping to decompress them)

2 Hang and bring one leg upwards as if hitching your hip into your waist, keeping your trunk vertical and your knees straight; then let that side go down as you bring the other side upwards. Repeat 5–20 times.
(Strengthens the side flexor muscles of the spine, especially quadratus lumborum)

3 Hanging, swing your legs gently from side to side, keeping your knees together and without twisting your body . Repeat 5–20 times. *(Mobilizes the low back)*

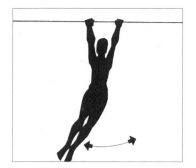

4 Hanging, keeping your trunk straight, gently part your legs, hold for a count of two, then slowly return to the starting position. Repeat 5–20 times. *(Strengthens your hip abductor muscles)*

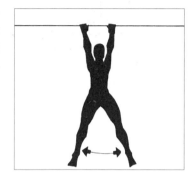

5 Hanging, bend one knee up to your chest, straighten the leg down again, take it slightly behind your body and then back to the starting position; then repeat the movement with the other leg. Do this 5–20 times.
(Strengthens and mobilizes the hip and pelvic muscles on the moving side, while the other side works to provide stability)

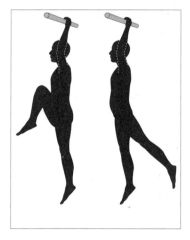

6 Hanging, bend both your knees up towards your chest, straighten your legs as you lower them, then take your legs slightly behind your body so that your back arches a little. Repeat 5–20 times.
(Strengthens your abdominal and back extensor muscles, and mobilizes your low back, pelvis and hips)

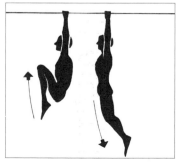

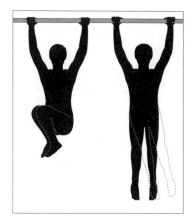

7 Hanging, bend both knees up towards your right shoulder, then lower them downwards, straightening and taking them slightly behind your body to the left; bring the knees up again, this time towards the left shoulder, and straighten them down so that they extend to the right behind you. Repeat 3–10 times.
(Strengthens the oblique abdominal muscles and the side flexor and rotator muscles of the back, while mobilizing the low back and hip regions)

8 Hanging, make small circles with your legs keeping your knees straight, right leg going clockwise, left anti-clockwise simultaneously. Repeat 3–10 times.
(Strengthens the muscles controlling your hips and pelvis)

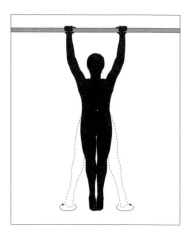

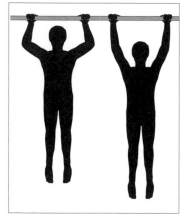

9 Hanging, bend your elbows to lift your bodyweight towards the bar, then slowly lower your body down again. Repeat 3–10 times without putting your feet on the floor.
(Strengthens latissimus dorsi especially, as well as chest, abdominal and back muscles)

Health, fitness training and your back

10

Fitness training should be a combination of different activities which match your aims and needs. For general fitness as well as for most sports, you need aerobic fitness, speed, possibly anaerobic fitness, muscle strength and endurance, possibly muscle power, muscle flexibility and joint mobility. All the types of exercise you might choose to do for fitness training should be carefully analysed, so that you do the right things to prevent back problems or recurrences. If you already have a back problem, in some cases it may still be possible to do some physical exercise to maintain a general level of fitness, if you choose your activities with care and strictly follow the instructions of your practitioner.

A general fitness programme for good health should automatically include a good balance of activities to give you all the necessary elements. If you are training for competitive sport, your programme should of course be geared to your sport, but it should also include protective elements to train those body parts which are not used by the sport itself, plus elements designed to counteract any positively harmful effects the sport might have on the body. Fitness training should aim to make you fit not just for your sport, but also for injury prevention and recovery.

> The fitter you are overall, the less likely you are to suffer back pain or injuries

TRAINING FOR SPORTS

The concept that you should train for a sport simply by practising that sport as much and as often as you can is very outdated. Some sports, such as horse-riding and pistol or rifle shooting, do very little for your physical fitness and health. Most sports carry the risk of overuse injuries, especially those involving repetitive patterns of movement, such as running, swimming, archery, canoe racing and rowing. In sports which carry the risk of traumatic injuries, such as show-jumping, skiing and contact events, you are more likely to recover fully and quickly from injuries if you have good basic body condition, beyond what is needed for the sport itself.

Physical training is just as important for the wheelchair athlete as it is for the able-bodied person. Sports involving repetitive, powerful movements, such as archery and the throwing events, can cause harmful rotational stresses on the upper part of the body. These must be counteracted with protective exercises and movements designed to make the body work in the opposite direction, to avoid pain in the spinal joints or shoulders.

The aims of fitness training

- to improve physical fitness, efficiency and health
- to improve performance in sports
- to improve co-ordination and neuromuscular efficiency
- to improve muscle strength, power and flexibility
- to improve joint mobility
- to improve cardiorespiratory efficiency
- to counteract the effects of repetitive stress due to sports
- to provide good body balance
- to help prevent sports-related injuries
- to prevent problems due to lack of physical fitness
- to help prevent degeneration effects due to disuse and ageing
- to assist recovery from any injuries

In sports involving a high degree of skill, such as tennis, golf, football and fencing, practice does not necessarily make perfect, mainly because a tired player tends to fall into bad habits, and is limited by existing physical deficits. On the other hand, if you extend your fitness parameters through a well-balanced training programme, your technical skills may improve together with your general fitness. The improvements in your speed and endurance will enhance your efficiency during the whole course of each game, match or competition, while your gains in flexibility and strength will allow you a greater variety of techniques or stroke production.

Both coaches and competitors have to be aware of what kind of training is relevant for the sport itself, and what is needed to provide good body balance for injury prevention.

THE WARM-UP AND WARM-DOWN

Every exercise session should start with a warm-up to prepare the body for physical activity. The warm-up makes the body work more efficiently. Whether it also prevents certain types of injury is not certain. The warm-down (or cooldown) is also very important, and it probably does help prevent muscle injuries through loosening the muscles which have been working and so preventing them from remaining tight and stiff. Pre-teen children do not necessarily need a warm-up and warm-down before and after energetic sports, but they are useful disciplines to instil early, as they become essential from the teenage years onwards.

Both the warm-up and the warm-down should consist of several parts, including controlled muscle stretching, mobilizing exercises, dynamic exercises to raise the pulse rate and cause some sweating, and perhaps some simulated skill practices in the warm-up for a sports match or competition. The warm-up should last at least fifteen minutes, and preferably longer, while the warm-down can be shorter, perhaps lasting ten minutes.

If you have suffered back or neck problems, it is useful to incorporate protective exercises within your warm-up and warm-down routines.

FLEXIBILITY AND MOBILITY TRAINING

I use the term 'flexibility' to apply to muscle length and pliability, and 'mobility' to refer to the freedom of movement in a joint. Your overall suppleness depends on both muscle and joint freedom. Good levels of flexibility and mobility are essential for healthy body condition. Having tight, short, strong muscles (being 'muscle bound') restricts the movements of your joints, and this can create compressive and shearing stresses in the spinal joints. Natural flexibility and mobility vary between individuals. In general, females are more flexible than males, Orientals more so than Caucasians.

During the body's normal bone growth phases there are periods when the muscles become relatively tight and weak, especially as the long bones of the legs grow. This is especially noticeable during the early teens, and again in the mid-teens, in both males and females. Adult males can lose overall body suppleness significantly as their muscular strength increases. Hormone changes in females, for instance in relation to the menstrual cycle or pregnancy, can cause a certain amount of muscle tightness, especially in the calves and the low back. Injury, disease and degeneration due to the effects of ageing are other factors which can reduce the natural range of movement in one's joints.

Sports like gymnastics and the martial arts are based on full body conditioning, and cultivate excellent muscle flexibility and joint mobility combined with muscle strength. If you do a sport which involves more limited patterns of movement, the chances are that you will have areas of muscle tightness and perhaps joint stiffness, unless you do training to compensate. Suppling exercises are used to make the body more pliable. They include techniques for improving joint mobility and muscle flexibility, which can be categorized as stretching and mobilizing exercises.

Stretching techniques

The safest and most efficient way to improve muscle flexibility is to do stretching exercises. In order to stretch a muscle group passively, the muscles have to be held still at their full length without pain or undue pressure. I prefer holding the stretch for a count of six, then relaxing completely before repeating it. Some people recommend holding a stretch for much longer, perhaps one minute or more, but this might lead to over-stretching if you lose concentration or try to increase the stretch from the already stretched position.

Apart from passive stretching, it is also possible to improve muscle flexibility using isometric contractions with the muscle group held at full length, followed by total relaxation. This is an active muscle stretching technique which is called 'hold-relax' and is part of a rehabilitation system for joint-muscle co-ordination called proprioceptive neuromuscular facilitation (PNF for short). Using this technique to increase length in the hamstring muscles, for instance, you sit on the floor with one leg straight in front of you, the other tucked out of the way; keeping your back straight and head up, lean forwards from the hips until you feel a gentle stretch; press the straight leg firmly against the floor for a count of three, relax completely, then lean forwards a little more from the hips. This type of active stretch can also be done with a partner providing resistance against the working muscles, with due care on both sides.

Stretching exercises are self-limiting, and should always be done within a comfortable range. Your muscles will be more pliable at times, for instance when you are warm, or after exercise. They will be tighter first thing in the morning and when you are cold. Provided you are aware of the muscle groups' elastic limits, you can do stretching exercises at any time without danger of injury through over-stretching.

Joint mobilizing techniques

Joint mobility exercises are usually performed as rhythmical bouncing movements. As you work through a joint's full range of movements you increase the flow of fluids through the joint, lubricating the joint surfaces. The tissues around the joint become more pliable as well, although the muscles around the joint do not necessarily stretch out in the same way as they do through passive or active stretching techniques.

Joint mobility can also be increased through passive techniques applied by another person. Most forms of manipulation and mobilization for the body's moving joints achieve an increase in range of movement, although this may be only temporary if it is not backed up with suitable exercises to maintain the new freedom of movement.

Protecting the spinal joints

To protect the back and neck, you have to be careful not to force any increase in muscle length or joint mobility. If you push too hard into a stretch or a mobilizing exercise, you are likely to go beyond the elastic limits of the joint structures, which might cause tearing. This is especially important when you are trying to increase mobility in the spinal joints themselves, or in closely related joints like the hips. In fact, in the adult it is quite difficult to increase the range in the spinal joints without running the risk of over-stretching and creating potentially harmful instability. The situation is similar during growth spurts, especially during the teenage years, when forceful mobilizing exercises can easily cause injury.

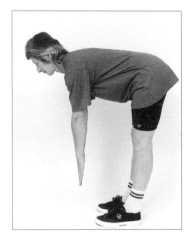

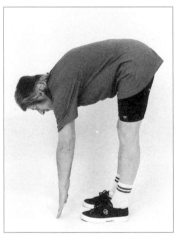

The hamstrings limit the forward tilt of the pelvis (*top*)
Even with relatively short hamstrings, it is still possible to touch the floor by over-stretching part of the spine (*bottom*)

Toe-touching is an example of a potentially dangerous mobility exercise which carries special risks for the back. It used to be considered an essential movement proving that you had good body condition, especially flexibility. If you could not touch your toes, you were encouraged to try your hardest to do so. In fact, forced toe-touching carries a strong risk of over-stretching and damaging the back. If you cannot touch your toes, there is no good reason to force the movement, and every reason not to.

If you have a problem in your back or neck, you may still be able to do some stretching and mobilizing exercises. However, you have to be careful not to put pressure on the spinal joints, especially through forward bending movements. Any stretching or mobilizing exercises involving the spinal joints should only be done under the direction of your practitioner. You may be prescribed movements like the 'slump' (sitting up and bending your head, neck and back) or the Yoga 'Cobra' stretch (lying on your stomach and lifting your upper body up resting your weight on your hands) to help your particular problem.

More generalized stretching and mobilizing exercises might be limited by your back pain. For instance, you may be unable to stretch your hamstrings sitting on the floor with your legs straight, but it might be possible to do so standing up by placing one leg on a low support in front of you, then bending forwards very slightly from the hips, keeping your back straight and head up (see p.194). Exercises involving the hips, such as seated adductor stretches and the standing splits, might be too painful. If you cannot find painfree alternatives, you must reduce or stop your suppleness programme until your spinal problem is cured.

AEROBIC, ANAEROBIC AND SPEED TRAINING

Aerobic exercise involves the efficient use of oxygen between the cardiorespiratory system and the working muscles. The lungs take in oxygen, the blood absorbs oxygen from the lungs, the heart pumps the blood to the working muscles, and the muscles use the oxygen in order to release energy. Stamina, or general endurance, is the ability to keep up aerobic exercise at quite a high rate over a space of time.

Anaerobic energy, by definition, does not involve oxygen, but mainly glycogen, which is stored in the muscle cells and is used by the working muscles when they cannot gain enough fuel from the aerobic (oxygen) sources. You use anaerobic energy for short sprints. Anaerobic work also comes into longer endurance events like canoeing when you put in intermittent bursts of speed.

Aerobic training is usually done as steady-state exercise taken at a reasonable pace, not flat-out. A session lasts at least twenty minutes but can continue for a lot longer, for instance if you are training for the marathon or long-distance cycling. Running, cycling, rowing, canoeing, cross-country skiing and brisk walking can all be used for aerobic training, whether in their natural forms or in the artificial versions using machines like treadmills and exercise bicycles. The exercise system called 'aerobics' was designed to improve cardiorespiratory fitness, and a typical aerobics session includes an extended period of jogging or jumping on the spot. The 'step class' is another popular type of aerobic training session. Repetitive aerobic training sessions carry a strong risk of overuse injuries, so they should not be done on consecutive days, and should be limited to three sessions a week.

Anaerobic training is usually done as intervals of high-intensity activity with short rest periods in between. Sprints, shuttle runs, or any exercise or combination of exercises can be used. The interval burst might be thirty seconds long, with a rest of thirty seconds. Progression might be to increase gradually the number of exercise bursts, and then to make the work time longer by stages, up to forty-five seconds. If you are doing a balanced training programme consisting of different types of exercise, the anaerobic session is usually done last within a day's exercise programme, and is generally limited to two sessions a week.

Speed training is also high-intensity activity in short bursts, but with a much longer rest phase, to avoid the build-up of lactic acid which is a by-product of the anaerobic energy system. For instance, the exercise interval can be as little as ten seconds, with a fifty-second pause between workout bursts. One way of combining speed and strength training is through *plyometrics*, a system which uses rapid bouncing or jumping movements to improve power through rhythmic repeated movements which work the muscles eccentrically and concentrically in quick succession. A session of plyometric drills might consist of sets of five or ten jumps repeated four to eight times at different heights. Plyometric sessions are usually limited to twice a week at most within a more generalized training programme.

Protecting the back and neck

Fitness training may involve repetitive activities such as running, so it is important to remember to safeguard the spinal joints, first by using protective exercises within the warm-up and warm-down, and second, by minimizing jarring and shearing stresses. For instance, if you run outside try to vary your running surface, and use simple but supportive shoes with protective cushioning insoles. Avoid excessive hill, camber or bend running, to prevent excessive pressure through the hips and pelvic joints. If you use a treadmill, wear simple indoor sports shoes, if possible with cushioning insoles. On a bicycle, make sure the saddle is high enough to let your knees straighten as you push down, but not so high that you have to tilt your pelvis sideways as each leg stretches downwards. If you row or use a rowing machine, learn the correct technique, so that you avoid faults such as 'bum-shoving', which puts the low back under extra stress.

When you are training at speed, choose exercises which are simple to do, especially if they involve machines. Otherwise you could fall off the machine, or start the exercise incorrectly.

If you have a back problem, you will probably be unable to do plyometric training without increasing your pain, because of the jarring forces. However, you may still be able to do aerobic, anaerobic and speed training by modifying your normal pattern of movement, or using different types of exercise. For instance, if you use a step machine, you may find it painful to use if you have to lean forwards on to the support bars, but perfectly comfortable if you can turn the other way and lean backwards with your spine supported while your legs work. With some types of back pain, you may not be able to use a rowing ergometer, but you might be able to substitute an Airdyne bicycle or its equivalent, where you are still using your arms and legs, but not directly involving your back.

If you find you cannot use your normal exercises for fitness training without pain, you may be able to construct a comparable programme using different machines or exercises. For general fitness and good body condition as a background for sports, it is best to train the whole body, not just

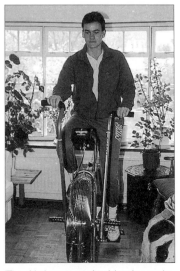

The Airdyne exercise bicycle works both the legs and arms aerobically

the parts you can see in the mirror, or that you need specifically for your sport. The greater the variety of your activities, the better your body condition, and the better your protection against injuries.

Tips for planning a safe and healthy training programme

- Make sure your programme is well balanced with a wide variety of activities and exercises
- Aim for good body conditioning, not just sport-specific fitness
- Include protective exercises for the back and neck in your warm-up and warm-down routines
- Avoid any potentially dangerous exercises
- Modify your programme or exercises according to any pain reactions
- Avoid any activities which you know cause or aggravate your spinal pain
- Never train through injury or illness
- Avoid overtraining: allow time each week for rest and relaxation
- Always be guided by your practitioner as to when to train and what type of exercise to do

---

WEIGHT TRAINING FOR STRENGTH, POWER AND FITNESS

Weight training is probably the most efficient method of improving strength, power and local muscle endurance. Strength is defined technically as the ability of a muscle to generate force. Power is the combination of muscle force with speed of movement. Muscle endurance allows a muscle to perform an action repetitively. A weight-training programme can also be used to improve aerobic fitness. As weightlifting or powerlifting, weight training can be done for its own sake; it can be used for bodybuilding, to create a bulky muscular physique; or it can be tailored as a general fitness programme. It is relevant to virtually all sports.

Adult males are, by definition, stronger than females,

although at certain stages of development during childhood females may be stronger than males of equivalent age. However both males and females can improve their basic strength through weight training, so there is no reason to identify weight training as a male preserve. A negative side of weightlifting, powerlifting and bodybuilding can be the use of anabolic steroids and similar drugs for artificial increases in muscle strength and bulk. Given the serious harmful effects these drugs can have, including liver and heart damage, anyone tempted to use them in relation to sports training should think twice. If you are determined to take this type of drug, seek guidance from a registered physician, not merely the 'pusher' promoting the latest drug cocktail in the local gym.

Weight training is important background conditioning work for sports, whether you play casually, seriously or competitively. Most sports require muscle endurance, strength and power in some mixture. Sprinting, competitive weightlifting, powerlifting and baseball require predominantly explosive power, whereas gymnastics and archery require strength. Endurance events include marathon and cross-country running, long-distance swimming and cycling, and cross-country skiing. In sports like volleyball, American football, rugby and basketball the player's position in the team may dictate the balance of strength, power and aerobic fitness required.

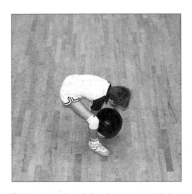

Background training is an essential discipline, but must be appropriate: young sports players should not be allowed to lift heavy weights incorrectly

Types of weight training

A weight-training programme consists of movements performed against a resistance. The resistance can be 'free weights', involving barbells and dumb-bells and discs specifying their weight in pounds or kilograms. 'Fixed-weights systems' use different types of resistance such as weight stacks, cords and pulleys, or weights and chains arranged with a cam system. These include Nautilus, Norsk, David, Schnell, and Sportesse. Some systems, like Hydrafitness, work with hydraulic resistance. You can use your own bodyweight as the resistance in exercises such as press-ups, chinning to a bar, hand-stands, head-stands and squats.

Most people do weight training in a gymnasium, with other people who can act as spotters, supervisors and motivators. It is also possible to do weight training at home, using simple free weights or home exercise weights equipment. To do this safely, you must be sure you know what you are doing, so you should have learned the principles and techniques from a qualified instructor. You should also ensure that the environment is safe, with enough space to move the weights around easily, and enough room to perform each exercise without hindrance. If you train alone, you should never take risks with very heavy weights, in case you cannot cope and have to drop the weight.

All exercises involving movement are called *dynamic* or *isotonic* exercises. When a muscle group shortens and contracts against gravity or a resistance, the contraction is termed *concentric*. The opposite movement, when a muscle group lengthens out, controlling a movement under the influence of a load or gravity, is called *eccentric*. You can also increase your strength *isometrically* or *statically* by pressing against an immovable resistance. You can incorporate isometric work into a dynamic exercise programme by holding the position still for a few seconds at the end of a movement.

Isokinetic muscle work is a contraction at a constant velocity, with the working muscles producing a variable force as they work through the range of the movement. The very sophisticated systems, such as the Kin-Com, Lido or Cybex, offer a variety of muscle work programmes, as well as the facility for computerized muscle measurements during joint movements including those of the back.

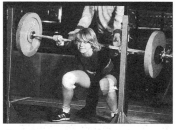

Close spotting is essential in case the lifter cannot manage a heavy weight

It is possible to incorporate cardiorespiratory training into a weight-training programme if you choose the right exercises and use the right equipment. You need to be able to do individual exercises at speed, within a circuit of exercises lasting at least half an hour overall. Each exercise can be done to a time span, such as twenty seconds, with an interval of perhaps ten seconds, or you can do fixed repetitions, perhaps fifteen or twenty of each exercise.

Weight-training programmes

Many weight-training exercises have special names, such as the *power clean*, *bench press*, *military press*, and the '*good morning*' exercise. Some are named according to the main muscle group they exercise, such as the *biceps curl*, *hamstring curl*, *latissimus pull*, and *triceps pull* or *triceps push*. Each complete movement in a particular exercise is termed a *repetition*. If you do a certain number of repetitions as a cycle of movements, this is called a *set*. You may have a fixed number of repetitions to do within each set, and a target of so many sets to do within one weight-training session. For endurance training, a customary pattern is to use relatively light weights to do three sets of fifteen or twenty repetitions, pausing to rest or to do other exercises between each set. For pure strength or power training, very heavy weights are lifted, pushed or pulled, not more than three times. The heaviest weight that you can move just once in any given exercise is technically known as your *one-repetition-maximum.*

The load you work against may vary according to the way the exercise is set up, or the type of machine you are using. For instance, lifting or pushing a weight upwards directly against the effect of gravity provides greater resistance than moving the same weight using a double pulley and cord system. Therefore moving a 100kg (220lbs) weight on a seated leg-press machine is much easier than pushing the same weight up with your legs working against a vertical stack. If you change from one type of system to another, do not try to do the same weights as previously. Play safe and start with much lighter weights than normal, then gradually build up the load as you get used to the new system.

All weight-training programmes should be progressive, so that you are aiming to achieve more over a space of time. Progression can involve increasing the weight resistance with each exercise, increasing the number of repetitions or sets of each exercise, timing each exercise and increasing the speed at which you perform the movements, increasing the number of different exercises you include within each session, or a combination of these parameters. A good weight-training programme should be constructed over the space of at least twelve weeks, as it takes about that long for muscles to adapt to a training programme. Training using exercises for the whole body should be done two or three times a week. If possible, the programme should last for sixteen weeks, after which there should be a break, and then a new programme devised.

The Norsk Sequence-Training System was designed for good body conditioning: within five basic exercises it provides muscle work through full range for all the body's major muscle groups. Because the exercises are simple to perform, and the machines easy to adjust, it is possible to use the system as circuit training for groups of individuals of very mixed abilities, including bodybuilders, professional sports competitors, and unfit people who have never done any kind of physical training before. The system has a particular value for people with ankylosing spondylitis (see p. 146).

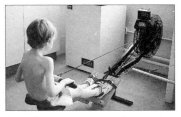

A rowing ergometer can be used for aerobic training. To use it correctly, you should straighten your legs as you pull the handle towards your stomach, leaning backwards slightly as your hands reach your body; then straighten your arms to take the handle over your knees before bending your knees and going forwards on the machine ready for the next stroke

In developing my own rehabilitation gymnasium, I have combined the basic Norsk system with other machines, such as the Hydrafitness step-machine, the Concept 2 rowing ergometer, mini-trampolines (PT Bouncers), the Hydrafitness Total Power and hip abduction/adduction machines, and grip exercisers, to provide different types of muscle, joint and cardiorespiratory work within the exercise circuit. People who have trained using the circuit have included, among others, Olympic competitors, young mothers, children with asthma and postural problems, people with arthritic conditions, countless back sufferers, and one of the longest-surviving heart transplant patients. Over fifteen years, there have been no accidents or injuries caused by the equipment or the exercise programme. An early study proved the benefits of the basic training programme, and virtually everyone who has trained regularly and consistently has reported both subjective and objective improvements in overall and localized fitness.

A well-constructed weight-training programme, properly done, can be invaluable in helping to prevent, alleviate or even cure certain types of spinal problem. However, weight-training exercises which are chosen badly or performed incorrectly can aggravate spinal problems, or in some cases actually cause them. Therefore, you have to be aware of the disadvantages and safety measures applicable to weight training in order to gain maximum benefit from it.

Dangers of weight training

1. Overload
If you try to lift, push or pull a weight which is beyond your strength, you risk injuring not only the working muscles and joints, but also any other parts of your body which are not properly supported or protected. This is especially dangerous for children and teenagers, who may *appear* capable of using heavier weights than their bodily maturity can really cope with.

2. Poor technique
The lifting technique for most free-weights exercises is complicated and has to be learned properly. Each movement has to be executed perfectly every time. Carelessness in handling the weights when you are setting up an exercise or tidying the weights away is one of the easiest ways to get injured. Incorrect lifting and handling almost inevitably lead to injury.

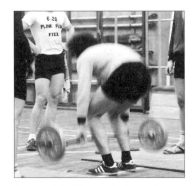

Poor weightlifting technique: the back should be straight and the knees fully bent to lift a heavy weight from the floor

3. Incorrect starting positions

Starting positions for free-weights exercises include sitting, standing, lying on your back, lying on your stomach and lying on your side. Choosing the wrong starting position for a movement is a common error. Another mistake, which can also happen if you use fixed-weight machines, is to have too little support for the parts of the body which are not involved in the actual exercise. This is the case if you stand up to do arm exercises, if the bench you lie on is too short, or if you use a seat with no back or with a backrest which does not support the head. Insufficient support leaves room for 'trick movements' and 'cheating', which can cause dangerous unwanted stresses in the body.

4. Poor exercise positioning

Whatever the starting position for a particular exercise, the weights bar, footplates or handles have to be positioned so that you can safely reach them and move them between the starting and finishing positions. Using free weights, your choice of exercises is restricted by the practical difficulties of combining correct starting positions with appropriate directions of movement against gravity. Weights machines allow a greater variety of movements against appropriate resistance, many of which cannot be simulated using free weights. When you use fixed-weights machines, you need to make sure that you adopt the correct position for every exercise, according to instructions.

5. Training alone

A spotter, or preferably two, should always be available to monitor free-weights exercises and to take the weight if you suddenly cannot manage it and fail in mid-lift. As I once lay for an hour trapped under a weights bar which had fallen across my chest while I was bench pressing, I can vouch for the need for spotters! The risk of dangerous overload is much less with fixed-weights machines, but you should nonetheless always be careful to learn correct use of the machines if you try an unfamiliar system.

6. Unbalanced training programmes

Using free weights, it is quite difficult to construct an all-round programme to create good body balance. It is hard to set up safe and efficient positions for isolating different muscle groups, especially in the back. It is easier to do heavy weightlifting using exercises which involve the front of the

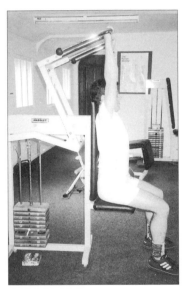

The Norsk pull-down machine: the spine is fully supported for this movement which strengthens all the major trunk muscles from a fully stretched position

trunk and arms. It is also the case of course that the front of the upper body is the part which is easiest to see in the mirror, if an athlete is looking out for muscle development. Bodybuilders in particular tend to concentrate on the quadriceps, abdominal, pectoral and biceps muscle groups, as they are the easiest to 'bulk up'.

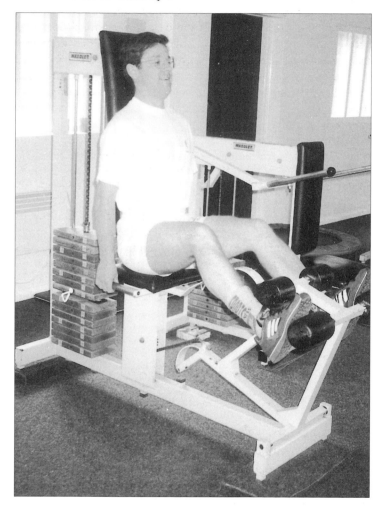

The Norsk leg-press machine. The whole spine is supported by the backrest, which is inclined backwards to prevent undue stress on any part of the spine during the movement of the hips and legs

Many people who train with free weights or machines, whether for fitness, bodybuilding or competitive weightlifting, do more exercises for the front half of the body than for the back. This can result in potentially harmful body imbalance. This kind of body imbalance might be especially dangerous to young weightlifters during the teenage growth spurts, as it affects their posture as young adults, and can lead to early or severe degenerative changes as they pass through middle age.

Weight training and protection for the back and neck

The safest way to do weight training of any kind is to use the modern systems which provide a machine as a station for each movement. Each machine should offer full support for all parts of the body which are not involved in the exercise, and a good range of movement against a resistance for the exercise itself. Some modern machines are designed to allow wheelchair athletes to use them. Otherwise people with paraplegia or other physical disabilities make use of free weights or pulley systems, doing the exercises sitting or lying down.

If you use free weights, you have to take care to train under safe conditions, to select a good range of exercises, to perform each exercise absolutely correctly, and to avoid possible harmful movements. Handling the weights correctly, even in between exercises, is absolutely essential. You should always keep your back as straight as possible when lifting even the lightest weight. For handling or lifting heavy weights, most weightlifters use a thick strong belt, which helps to reinforce correct trunk posture, not least by reminding them to keep their back straight. When lifting heavy weights off the floor in exercises such as the deadlift, snatch or power clean, lifters usually take in a deep breath and block the exhalation, holding their breath in forcibly. Called *Valsalva's manoeuvre*, this technique raises the pressure in the abdominal and thoracic cavities, and very slightly reduces the pressure within the intervertebral discs in the low back.

Standing and leaning forwards with even a light load places potentially excessive pressure on your lower back, even if you have never had any back problems. Unfortunately, some free-weights exercises which are accepted as standard in weight-training manuals, are potential disasters for the back, because they ignore this basic rule. One example is the 'good morning' exercise. For this, you stand with a weights bar across your shoulders behind your neck, bend over forwards from the hips, then straighten up again. The stress on the low back intensifies the longer you hold the position isometrically while you perform the repetitions in each set. The bent-over rowing exercise is another

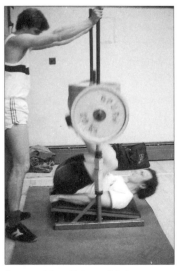

Free weights: if the pelvis is not directly under the weights stack in the lying leg press, the low back muscles are also used to push the weights up. If the head is not supported, the spine is stressed from the upper end as well.

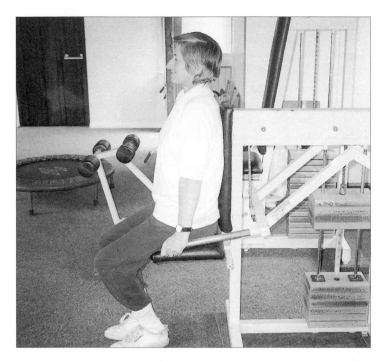

The Norsk dip machine: the back is well supported for this exercise which stretches the chest and upper back muscles before they contract to push the machine's handles down. Like all the Norsk machines, this one provides good balance between different muscle groups.

example. You stand and lean forwards with your arms straight down and a weights bar in your hands, then you lift the bar towards your chest, and lower it down again. Both these exercises would be better done lying on your stomach. To simulate the 'good morning' exercise and strengthen the back muscles, you should lie over the edge of a bench with your feet fixed and perhaps a very light weight behind your neck. The substitute for bent-over rowing is to lie on a high bench and pull the weights bar from the floor towards your chest.

Cheating is a general risk in any kind of weight training. It creates extra and unwanted stresses on the body, even though it can be tempting to try to lift, push or pull heavier weights than you really can or should. For instance, the 'biceps curl' movement, done standing up, allows you to bend and straighten your back, bringing in extra strength through your trunk muscles, as you straighten and bend your elbows to move the weight or dumb-bells between your thighs and your shoulders. In any kind of leg-press movement, where you press the soles of your feet against the footplate supporting the weight resistance, and straighten your knees, you can recruit the seat muscles (gluteals) as strength reinforcement.

This is done by bending the hips and curving the lower back, and can happen whether the leg press is done lying on your back or sitting up, with a weights stack or on a fixed-weights machine. The bench-press exercise is done lying on the back, whether using free weights, a pulley system or using a weights machine; the weights bar is pushed vertically upwards from across the chest, then slowly lowered down again. If the weight is very heavy for you, arching your back to bring the back muscles into play provides more strength for the movement.

To prevent cheating and to protect the back, all the non-working parts of the body should be totally supported, and you should be properly placed in relation to the supporting surfaces. For exercises done sitting up, your back and head should be fully supported on a vertical or backward slanted backrest. For the bench press and other arm exercises done lying on your back, your knees should be bent and your feet supported on the bench, or on a chair or extension placed at the end of it, if the bench itself is too short. For stomach-lying exercises, such as the hamstring curl, you should place a cushion under your hips to reduce the pressure on your back, if the bench is not shaped to hold your hips slightly bent. If you use a vertical leg-press machine or weights stack, you must make sure that your bottom is vertically under the foot-plate, so that your legs extend in parallel with the support struts of the machine.

Some weight-training exercises place compressive loads on the spinal joints, and are therefore unsuitable if you have a back problem. Lifting weights up above your head when you are upright, whether sitting or standing, places great stress on your neck and your lower back, so this type of exercise should certainly be avoided if you have any stiffness or pain in these regions. The seated military press is especially compressive for the lowest part of the back. Whether you use a free-weights bar, dumb-bells, or a pulley machine system, as you push the load upwards above your head, all the force of the weight plus the effect of gravity are transmitted to the lowest part of your back, without any dissipation, as the downward force is met by an equal and opposite pressure directly under your seat. If your back is not properly supported, you run the further risk of shifting your trunk slightly awkwardly and injuring yourself as you perform the lift.

Squats done with the weights bar behind your neck are also very compressive on the spine, especially if you use very heavy weights. Holding the bar behind your head also pushes your head forwards, which creates pressure on the neck joints. The neck is also subjected to unwanted strain when you pull the bar down behind your neck for the 'lats pull-down' exercise, which is done using a fixed-weights machine or pulley system. The squat exercises can be modified to reduce the pressure on the spinal joints by holding the bar in front of the chest or using dumb-bells in the hands. For the lats pull-down the bar can be brought down in front of the body, so that the head can be held up throughout the movement.

Problem prevention checklist

- Develop and cultivate good postural habits from the earliest age
- Keep to a regular, healthy diet, and drink plenty of plain water
- Do protective exercises for the back, neck and whole body systematically and frequently
- Take regular exercise for general health
- Do fitness training as background for your sport
- Develop good balance between related joints and muscle groups
- Cultivate good muscle flexibility and strength
- Always lift any kind of load or object safely and correctly
- Set aside time each day for rest and relaxation
- Regulate your lifestyle to avoid or minimize harmful physical or mental stresses

When planning to use a weight-training programme, you must be sure that you know exactly how to achieve your aims safely. You may need instruction in techniques, even for the simplest-looking exercise machines. Monitoring by a fitness instructor prevents carelessness during exercise sessions. In a properly regulated gymnasium, there should always be a responsible person supervising, who is not only experienced in exercise instruction, but is also qualified to perform basic first-aid. The instructor should be sensitive to people's individual capacities and problems during training, and should never contradict advice on exercise or technique given to a client by a qualified practitioner.

If you have problems with your back or neck, you should take advice from your practitioner as to whether to train, or which exercises to do. If your fitness instructor is in doubt as to whether it is safe for you to train, you may be able to arrange for your physiotherapist to explain the details of what you should or should not do. Your physiotherapist might even attend the gymnasium with you to check on your exercise performance and modify your programme, preferably in conjunction with your fitness instructor, if you have one.

Recommended reading

BOOKS AND MANUALS

Those which are suitable for non-professional readers are marked with an asterisk

*Andrews, E, 1991, *Muscle Management*, Thorsons

Arnold, L E, 1978, *Chiropractic Procedural Examination*, Seminole Printing Inc., Florida

Baldry, P E, 1993, *Acupuncture, Trigger Points and Musculoskeletal Pain*, Churchill Livingstone, Edinburgh, 2nd Edition

Bergmann, T F, Peterson D H, Lawrence D J, 1993, *Chiropractic Technique*, Churchill Livingstone, Edinburgh

Bogduk, N, Twomey, L T, 1987, *Clinical Anatomy of the Lumbar Spine*, Churchill Livingstone, Melbourne, Edinburgh

Bourdillon, J F, Day, E A, 1987, *Spinal Manipulation*, Heinemann Medical Books, Oxford, 4th Edition

Boyling, J D, Palastanga, N, (Eds) 1994, *Grieve's Modern Manual Therapy: The Vertebral Column*, Churchill Livingstone, Edinburgh, 2nd Edn

* Brennan, R, 1992, *The Alexander Technique Workbook*, Element, Shaftesbury UK

Bromley, I, 1991, *Tetraplegia and Paraplegia: A Guide for Physiotherapists*, Churchill Livingstone, Edinburgh, 4th Edn

* Burn, L, Paterson J, 1993, *Back Pain. A handbook for sufferers*, Headway: Hodder and Stoughton, Sevenoaks, Kent UK

Byfield, D, (Ed) 1995, *Chiropractic Manipulative Skills: The Fundamentals of Clinical Practice*, Butterworth Heinemann, London

* Chaitow, L, 1983, *The Acupuncture Treatment of Pain*, Thorsons, London, 2nd Edition

* Coplands-Griffiths, M, 1991, *Dynamic Chiropractors Today*, Thorsons, London

Corrigan, B, Maitland, G D, 1983, *Practical Orthopaedic Medicine*, Butterworths, London

Cyriax, J, 1982, *Textbook of Orthopaedic Medicine. Volume 1, Diagnosis of Soft Tissue Lesions*, Baillère Tindall, London, 8th Edition

Cyriax, J, 1984, *Textbook of Orthopaedic Medicine. Volume 2, Treatment by Manipulation, Massage and Injection*, Baillère Tindall, London

D'Orazio, B, (Ed) 1993, *Back Pain Rehabilitation*, Butterworth Heinemann, Oxford

DiGiovanna, E L, and Schiowitz, S, (Eds) 1991, *An Osteopathic Approach to Diagnosis and Treatment*, J B Lippincott company, Philadelphia

Donatelli, R A, Wooden, M J, 1994, *Orthopaedic Physical Therapy*, Churchill Livingstone, Edinburgh, 2nd Edn

Dvir, Z, 1995, *Isokinetics. Muscle Testing, Interpretation and Clinical Applications*, Churchill Livingstone International, New York

Edwards, B C, 1992, *Manual of Combined Movements*, Churchill Livingstone, Edinburgh

Glasgow, E F, Twomey, L T, Scull, E R, Kleynhans, A M, (Eds) 1985, *Aspects of Manipulative Therapy*, Churchill Livingstone, Edinburgh 2nd Edn

Greenman, P E, 1989, *Principles of Manual Medicine*, Williams and Wilkins, Baltimore

Grieve, G, 1988, *Common Vertebral Joint Problems*, Churchill Livingstone, 2nd Edn

Grieve, G, 1991, *Mobilisation of the Spine: A Primary Handbook of Clinical Method*, Churchill Livingstone, 5th Edn

Hartman, L S, 1990, *Handbook of Osteopathic Technique*, Unwin Hyman Ltd, London, 2nd Edition

Hayne, C R, 1987, *Total Back Care*, J M Dent & Sons, London and Melbourne

* Howat-Wilson, M B, 1991, *Chiropractic: A Patients' Guide*, Thorsons, London 2nd Edn

* Hutchinson, E T L, 1991, *Moving and Lifting for Carers*, Woodhead Faulkner

Hutson, M, 1993, *Back Pain, Recognition and Management*, Butterworth-Heinemann, Oxford

* Iyengar, B K S, 1968 *Light on Yoga*, Unwin Paperbacks, London

Janda, V, 1983, *Muscle Function Testing*, Butterworth, London

Jayson, M (Ed), 1980, *The Neurology of Low Back Pain*, Pitman Medical, Tunbridge Wells

Jayson, M I V, 1992, *The Lumbar Spine and Back Pain*, Churchill Livingstone, Edinburgh, 4th Edn

Kahn, J, 1994, *Principles and Practice of Electrotherapy*, Churchill Livingstone, Edinburgh

Kaltenborn, F, 1970, *Mobilization of the Spinal Column*, New Zealand University Press, Wellington

Kidd, G, Lawes, N, Musa, I, 1992 *Understanding Neuromuscular Plasticity*, A basis for clinical rehabilitation. Edward Arnold, London

Kirkaldy-Willis, W, H, Burton, C V, 1992, *Managing Low Back Pain*, Churchill Livingstone, Edinburgh, 3rd Edn

Lee, D, 1989, *The Pelvic Girdle*, Churchill Livingstone, Edinburgh

* Leibowitz, J, Connington, W, 1991, *The Alexander Technique*, Souvenir Press, London

Lewit, K, 1985, *Manipulative Therapy in Rehabilitation of the Locomotor System*, Butterworths, London

Low, J, Reed, A, 1994, *Electrotherapy Explained*, Butterworth Heinemann, London

* Macdonald, G, 1994, *Alexander Technique*, Headway: Hodder & Stoughton, Sevenoaks (UK)

Maitland, G D, 1986, *Vertebral Manipulation*, Butterworths, London, 5th Edn

McKenzie, R, 1981, *The Lumbar Spine, Mechanical Diagnosis and Therapy*, Spinal Publications Waikanae, New Zealand

* McKenzie, R, 1983, *Treat Your Own Neck*, Spinal Publications Waikanae, New Zealand

* McKenzie, R, 1983, *Treat Your Own Back*, Spinal Publications Waikanae, New Zealand

* Meadows-Smith, R, 1994, *Back to Health (Help for Back Problems)*, Available from: Cleve Lodge, 42 Warren Rd, Orpington, Kent BR6 5HY

Melzack, R, Wall, P D, 1982 *The Challenge of Pain*, Basic Books, New York

Mennell, J, 1952, *The Science and Art of Joint Manipulation*, Churchill Livingstone, London

Mennell, J, 1964, *Joint Pain*, Churchill Livingstone, London

* Moore, S, 1988, *New Ways to Health Series: A Guide To Chiropractic*, Hamlyn, London

Mulligan, B R, 1992, *Manual Therapy: NAGS, SNAGS and PRPs etc*, Plane View Services, Wellington NZ, 2nd edn

National Back Pain Association in collaboration with the Royal College of Nursing, 1992, *Guide to the Handling of Patients*, NBPA, London

Nicholas, J A, Hershman, E B, (Eds) 1986, *The Lower Extremity and Spine in Sports Medicine, Volumes 1 & 2*, C V Mosby Company, St Louis

* Nickel, D J, 1984, *Acupressure for Athletes*, An Owl Book, New York

Porter, R W, (Ed) 1994, *Management of Back Pain*, Churchill Livingstone, Edinburgh, 2nd Edn

Porterfield, J A, DeRosa, C, 1991, *Mechanical Low Back Pain: Perspectives in Functional Anatomy*, W B Saunders Co, Philadelphia

Reid, D C, 1992, *Sports Injury Assessment and Rehabilitation*, Churchill Livingstone, New York

* Saunders, H D, 1994, *Self-Help Manual – For your back*, The Saunders Group Inc, Chaska (US)

* Saunders, H D, 1994, *Self-Help Manual – For your neck*, The Saunders Group Inc, Chaska (US)

* Saunders, H D, 1994, *Self-Help Manual – Managing back pain*, The Saunders Group Inc, Chaska (US)

* Sharp, E, 1993, *The Healthy Back Book*, Elements, Shaftesbury, Dorset

* Sherwood, P, 1992, *The Back and Beyond*, Arrow, London

Skinner, A T, Thomson, A M, (Eds) 1983, *Duffield's Exercise in Water*, Baillière Tindall, London, 3rd Edn

Stoddard, A, 1993, *Manual of Osteopathic Practice*, Osteopathic Supplies Ltd

Stoddard, A, 1993, *Manual of Osteopathic Technique*, Osteopathic Supplies Ltd

Sutherland, W G, 1990, *Teachings in the Science of Osteopathy*, Rudra Press

Thie, J F, 1979, *Touch for Health*, De Vorss & Co, Marina del Rey, California, 2nd Edition

Twomey, L T, Taylor, J R, (Eds) 1994, *Physical Therapy of the Low Back*, Churchill Livingstone, Edinburgh, 2nd Edn

Upledger, J E, Vreedevoogd, J D, 1983, *Craniosacral Therapy*, Eastland Press, Seattle

Wells, P E, Frampton, V, Bowsher, D, (Eds) 1988, *Pain Management and Control in Physiotherapy*, Heinemann, London

Williams, P L, Bannister, L L, Berry, M, Collins, P, Dussek, J, Dyson, M, Ferguson, M W J, (Eds) 1995, *Gray's Anatomy*, Churchill Livingstone International, Edinburgh, 38th Edn

Index

Abdominal muscles, 4, 26, 57, 116,119, 134, 157, 158, 159, 175, 182, 213
Abdominal surgery, 6
Acrobatics, 9, 35
Acupressure, 105
Acupuncture, 67
Acupuncturist(s), 98, 151
Acute pain, 7, 88, 90
Adult(s), 15, 46, 99, 124, 139, 144, 207
'Adverse neural tension' (ANT), 111, 129
Aerobic fitness, training, 181, 199, 204–7
'Aerobics', 205
Age, ageing, 4, 6, 8, 42, 53, 132, 136, 147, 200
Airdyne bicycle, 206
Airport staff, 30
Alexander technique, 98
Allergies, 98
American Association of Orthopaedic Medicine, 106
American football, 8, 87, 130, 208
American Physical Therapy Association, 99
Anabolic steroids, 208
Anaerobic fitness, 199, 204–7
Anaesthetist, 97
Ankylosing spondylitis, 137, 146–7, 179, 210
Annulus fibrosus, 47, 70, 130, 132
Apophyses, 41

Apparent shortening (of the leg), 5, 140
Applied kinesiologist(s), 98
Archery, 12, 200, 208
Aromatherapist(s), 98, 151
Assessment, 94, 123–6
Asthma, 102
Athlete(s), 2, 109
Australian Physical Therapy Association, 99
Autonomic nervous system, 48

Baby, babies, 2, 26, 99
'Back chair', 20
Back extensor (erector spinae) muscles, 4, 58, 119, 136, 161, 162, 163, 164, 165, 166
Back School(s), 67
Badminton, 11
Baggage handlers, 30
Bags, 28–31
Balance, 9, 55, 116, 169
Baseball, 11, 172, 208
Basketball, 85, 208
Bath, 27, 35
Beautician(s), 35
Bed, 18, 27, 37, 90
Bed-making, 31
Bed-rest, 67, 118, 131, 139
Bed-wetting, 102
Biceps muscles, 5, 213
Biofeedback, 114, 150
Biomechanical tests, 127, 153
Blood flow, circulation, 17, 20, 100, 114, 141, 181

Blood pressure, 21, 102
Blood test(s), 94, 122, 147, 149, 152
Blood vessels, 39, 51, 70
Body balance, 3–7, 9
Body mechanics, 5, 13
Bodybuilding, 207, 213
Bodyweight, 9, 10
Bone growth, 40–1
Bone slippage (spondylolisthesis), 142–3
Bone(s), 39–44, 51, 52
'Bone-setters', 103
Bourdillon, Professor J, 108
Bowel motions, 65, 126, 131
Boxing, 87, 131
Brain, 48, 51, 52
Brain contusion, 87, 145
Breast-bone (sternum), 40, 51, 175
British Institute of Musculoskeletal Medicine, 106
Brittle bones (osteoporosis), 80, 132, 135, 147
Bronchitis, 149
Building work, 24
Butler, Mr David, 108

Calf muscle(s), 21
Canadian Physical Therapy Association 99
Cancer (malignant disease), 74, 81, 114, 147
Canoeing, 12, 200, 205
Car, 22–3, 89

Car accident(s), 7, 131, 141, 145, 153
Cardiorespiratory training, 209
Carer, 27, 35
Carrying, 24, 28–31
Cartilage, 40, 46–7
Cartilaginous joint(s), 44
Cauda equina, 49
Caudal epidural injection, 107
Central nervous system, 1, 48–51, 71, 98
Centre of gravity, 3
Centre of ossification, 40
Cerebrospinal fluid, 49
Cervical lordosis, 2
Chair(s), 17–21, 89
Chartered Society of Physiotherapy, 99
Chemonucleolysis, 113
Chest illness(es), 74
Chest physiotherapy, 99
Childbearing, 2
Childbirth, 6, 26, 36, 80, 81–2, 92
Childhood, 3, 41, 46, 47, 134
Childrearing, 83
Children, 15, 18, 28, 52, 68, 87, 99, 118, 125, 139, 143, 144, 149, 201, 211
Chiropodist(s), 35, 98
Chiropractic, 67, 101–2
Chiropractor, 93, 98, 100–2, 108
Chronic pain, 67-68, 101–2
Circulation (blood flow), 17, 20, 100, 114, 141
Clavicle (collar-bone), 54, 62
Clinical depression, 67, 75, 98
Clinical history, 124
Clinical psychologist, 98
Co-ordination, 5, 9, 49, 54, 55, 113–15, 116, 148, 157, 158, 159, 162, 200
Coach driver(s), 30
'Cobra' exercise, 204
Coccyx (tailbone), 39, 41, 43, 44, 49, 107
Collar (support for neck), 16, 87, 88, 137, 144, 145, 150
Collar-bone (clavicle), 54, 62
Colleges of Osteopathic Medicine, 102
Coma, 99

Combined movements, 110
Compensation, 3, 6, 13, 28, 140, 170
Competitive sport, 10, 201
Complementary practitioners, 98
Compression forces, 7, 9, 10, 23, 28, 72, 131, 183
Compression fracture, 133
Computer(s), 21
Computerized Axial Tomography (CAT, CT scans), 122, 149
Concentric muscle contraction, 55
Concept 2 rowing ergometer, 211
Concussion, 87
Contact sports, 87
Contraceptive pill, 36, 79–80
Cooking, 32-33
Cool-down (warm-down), 181, 201
Corset (support for back), 16, 88–9, 104, 133, 139, 144
Costovertebral joints, 46
Cough, 57, 59, 65, 131
Craniosacral therapy, 111
'Crick' in the neck (torticollis, 'wry neck'), 144–5
Cricket, 11, 87
Cricketers, 142, 172
Cross-country running, 208
Cross-country skiing, 60, 205, 208
Crutches, 3
Cumulative overuse strains, 13
Curves, curvature of the spine, 2, 3, 10, 16, 57, 59, 60, 131, 134, 139, 175
Cybex isokinetic machine, 209
Cycling, 12–13, 87, 142, 205, 208
Cyriax, Dr James, 106, 108

Dangerous exercises, 182–3, 204
David exercise system, 208
Decorating, 32, 92
Deltoid muscle(s), 171
Dentists, 35
Depression, 67, 75, 80, 98
Desk, 20–1
Diadynamic therapy, 114

Diagnosis, 69, 94, 121–3
Diet, 76–9, 81, 91, 126, 148, 153
Dietician, 98
Disc degeneration, 24, 47, 53, 70, 113, 135, 144
Disc problems, 94, 115, 130–2, 139, 149
Disc(s) (intervertebral), 7, 24, 39, 46–7, 49, 52, 53, 70, 94, 106, 109–13, 115, 130–2, 135, 139, 144, 149
Discectomy, 113
Discus thrower(s), 172
Disease, 8, 71, 121
Diving, 7, 141
Dizziness, 145
Do-it-yourself jobs, 32
Doctor(s), 1, 80, 93, 97, 106, 123, 156, 182
Dominant arm, 3, 4, 12
Double-leg-raising exercise, 182
'Dowager's hump', 3, 148
Dressing, 35–6
Driving, 22–3, 88, 125, 141
Drug dependence, 67
Drugs, 67, 88, 94, 101, 118, 131, 144, 149
Dynamic (isotonic) muscle work, 55, 209

Eccentric muscle contraction, 55, 209
Electrical muscle stimulation, 114, 115, 117, 140, 144, 145, 148
Electrotherapy, 99–101, 106, 113–15, 117, 132, 137
Employment, 15, 67
Endurance, 199, 207
Environment, 8, 27
Epidural injection, 82, 97, 107
Epiphyseal plate (growth plate, growth cartilage), 40, 138
Epiphysis, 40, 114
Equipment, 8
Erector spinae (back extensor) muscles, 4, 58, 119, 136, 161, 162, 163, 164, 165, 166
Ergonomics, 100
Exercise bicycle(s), 205, 206
Exercise breaks, 19, 23
Exercise tests, 153–78
Exercise therapy, 99, 115–17

Facet (zygapophyseal) joints, 42, 44, 45, 49, 53, 70, 132–33, 144
'Facet syndrome', 133
Family doctor (general practitioner, GP), 80, 81, 87, 88, 93, 97, 98, 101, 103, 151
Family life, 67
Fatigue, 8, 26, 75, 125
Fatigue (stress) fracture, 123, 142
Fear, 63, 66, 68, 75
Female(s), 9, 24, 36, 42, 51, 74, 77, 79–83, 92, 99, 126, 147, 202
Femoral nerve, 50, 72
Femoral nerve stretch test, 128
Fencing, 4, 45, 200
Fibrocartilaginous joint(s), 45
'Fibrositis', 94, 133
Fibula (outer leg-bone), 60
Field hockey, 54
First aid, 8, 85–7
Fitness training, 12, 199-218
Flank-bones (innominate bones, ilia), 39, 41, 43, 46
'Floating' rib(s), 40, 45, 46, 58
Flying, 9
Food intolerance, 76–9, 81, 98
Foot alignment, 4
Football (soccer), 5, 12, 200
Fracture(s), 123, 133–4, 142–4, 148
'Frozen shoulder', 77, 80
Frymann, Dr Viola, 108
'Functional techniques', 110

'g' forces, 9
Gardening, 25, 89–92
General practitioner (GP, family doctor), 80, 81, 87, 88, 93, 97, 98, 101, 103, 151
Glandular fever, 151–2
Gluteus muscles, 4, 44, 60, 161, 162, 163, 164, 178
Golf, 11, 137, 200
Gout, 137, 146
Gravity, 1, 2, 3, 10, 21, 58
Grieve, Mr Gregory, 108
Groin injury, 182
Growth, 4, 8, 14, 47, 153, 202, 203
Growth cartilage (growth plate, epiphyseal plate), 40, 138

Gymnast(s), 7, 9, 142
Gymnastics, 9, 10, 59, 85, 134, 140, 202, 208
Gynaecological problems, 74
Gynaecologist, 80

Hair washing, 34
Hairdresser(s), 35
Hammer throwing, 11
Hamstrings, hamstring muscles, 5, 44, 60, 161, 162, 163, 164, 174, 204
Handedness, 4
Hanging, 177, 181, 196–8
Harness (support for upper back), 16
Head, 1, 20, 42, 52, 71
Head injury, 48
Headache(s), 65, 76, 80, 87, 102, 121, 136
Healing, 67
Health, 92, 199
Heart, 48, 51
Hereditary condition(s), 74, 147, 148
Hernia, 182
Herniated disc, 130
High jump, 9
Hip abductor muscles, 60, 167, 168, 169
Hip adductor muscles, 172
Hip flexor muscles (iliopsoas), 43, 59
Hip(s), 4, 5, 7, 10, 12, 43–4, 59, 79, 146, 161, 162, 163, 164, 178
Hobbies, 18
'Hold-relax' technique , 202
Homeopath, 151
Hormonal influences, 2, 8, 26, 74, 77, 79–83, 92, 126, 137, 202
Hormone Replacement Therapy (HRT), 81–2, 92, 148
Horse riding, 8, 9, 87, 141, 199
Hospital treatment, 87, 111
Hot and cold treatments, 136
Housework, 31–3
Hunchback, 134, 139
Hydrafitness exercise system, 208, 211
Hydrotherapy (pool exercises), 99, 183–4

Hypermobile joint(s), 179
Hyperparathyroidism, 146
Hypomobile joint(s), 179

Ice hockey, 8
Ice therapy, 90, 123, 136
Idiopathic kyphosis, 134
Idiopathic scoliosis, 139
Ilia (flank-bones, innominate bones), 39, 41, 43, 46
Iliac crests, 44
Iliopsoas (hip flexor muscles), 43, 59
Illness(es), 8, 74, 92,125, 149–52, 180
Immobilization (after injury), 6
In-vitro-fertilization, 102
Infection(s), 67, 74, 92, 122, 125, 149–52, 180
Infective discitis, 149
Inflammation, 122, 149
Inflammatory bowel disorders, 146
Inflammatory diseases, problems, 146–9
Injection(s), 105, 107, 112
Innominate bones (flank-bones, ilia), 39, 41, 43, 46
Interferential therapy, 101, 114
International Federation of Orthopaedic Manipulative Therapists, 100
Intervertebral discs, 7, 24, 39, 46–7, 49, 52, 53, 70, 94, 106, 109–13, 115, 130–2, 135, 139, 144, 149
Intervertebral foramen, 44
Investigations, 93, 121
Irritable bowel syndrome, 102
Ischial tuberosity (seat-bone), 44, 60, 174
Isokinetic exercise (testing) equipment, 153, 209
Isometric (static) muscle work, 55, 209
Isotonic (dynamic) muscle work, 55, 209

Janda, Dr Vladimir, 108
Jarring stresses, 13, 41
Javelin, 11, 172
Joint capsule(s), 39
Joint distortion, 13

Joint mobility, stability and limitation(s), 53–4, 199, 203
Joint(s), 1, 44–7, 53
Jump(s), jumping events, 9, 60, 170

Kaltenborn, Dr Freddy, 108
Karate, 9
Kidney infections, 74
Kin-Com isokinetic machine, 209
'Kissing spines', 134
Knee problems, 164, 178
Kneeling, 1
Kyphosis, 3, 134, 138, 148

Lacrosse, 87
Laminectomy, 113
Laser therapy, 113
Latissimus dorsi muscle(s), 59, 62, 169
Leg alignment, 4
Leg length differences, 4, 5, 43, 98, 140
Levator scapulae muscle(s), 61
Leverage for movement, 50, 53–4
Lewit, Dr Karel, 108
Lido isokinetic machine, 209
Life-saving measures, 86
Lifting, 13, 14, 23–31, 67
Lifting technique, 14, 24, 211, 214–17
Ligament(s), 1, 7, 39, 45–6
Limp, 6
Line of gravity, 3
'Locked joint', 106, 107
Lordosis, 2, 3, 10, 57, 59, 60, 175
Lorry driver, 23
Low mood, 26, 75
'Lumbago', 94, 135
Lumbar lordosis, 2, 3, 10, 57, 59, 60, 175
Lumbar Motion Monitor
Lungs, 51
Lying down, 37, 65, 90, 125

Mackenzie, Mr Brian, 108
Magnetic resonance imaging (MRI), 113, 122, 134, 146, 149
Maitland, Mr Geoffrey, 108

Male(s), 10, 36, 59, 147, 207
Malignant disease (cancer), 74, 81, 114, 147
Manipulation(s), 87, 94, 100, 101, 102, 103, 105, 106, 107, 118, 136, 148, 203
Manipulation Association of Chartered Physiotherapists (MACP), 100
Manipulation under anaesthetic (MUA), 109
Manual therapy, 96, 99, 103, 105–6, 117, 132, 137, 139, 145
Manual work, 23–8, 136
Marathon runner, 151
Marathon running, 208
Martial arts, 202
Massage, 87, 99, 105, 106
Mechanical causes of spinal pain, 69–73, 121, 130–46
Median nerve, 50
Medical osteopath, 93
Medico-legal case(s), 153
Medulla spinalis (spinal cord, neuraxis), 48–50, 51
Menarche (onset of periods), 2
Meninges, 49
Mennell, Dr James, 108
Menopause, 2, 42, 77, 80–1, 92, 147
Menstruation (periods), 2, 79, 92, 202
Metabolic diseases, 146
Microdiscectomy, 113
Migraine(s), 102
Milk round, 24
Mini-trampolines (PT Bouncers), 211
Mobility, 199, 203
Mobilizations, 100, 105, 109–11, 135, 150, 203
Mobilizing exercises, 184, 185–93
Morning stiffness, 11, 65, 146
Motherhood, 26, 82–3, 116
Motor nerves, 48
Motor racing, 9, 87
Mouth-to-mouth resuscitation, 86
Mulligan, Mr Brian, 108
Multifidus muscles, 58
'Muscle bound', 201

'Muscle energy techniques', 110
Muscle flexibility, 199, 201–3
Muscle imbalance, 6, 10, 13, 62
Muscle power, 199, 207
Muscle relaxants, 67
Muscle spasm, 2, 6, 73, 90, 100, 105, 108, 109, 128, 135, 179
Muscle tone, 1, 2, 17, 75, 114, 128, 179
Muscle(s), 1, 7, 39, 54–62
Muscular inefficiency, 6
Musculoskeletal problems, 69–73
Myalgic encephalomyelitis (ME), 151
Myelogram(s), 94, 122

Nautilus exercise system, 208
Nerve disruption (neurological signs), 72, 115, 123
Nerve root compression, 72, 128, 131, 139, 180
Nerves, 39, 48–50, 64, 65, 71, 73
Neuraxis (spinal cord, medulla spinalis), 48–50, 51
Neurological signs (nerve disruption), 72, 115, 123
Neuromuscular co-ordination, 55, 113, 115
Neurosurgeon, 97, 113, 131
Newspaper round, 24, 29
Night pain, 66
Norsk exercise equipment, 25, 119, 120, 147, 208, 210–11, 212, 213, 215
Nucleus pulposus, 47, 70, 130
Nurse(s), 27, 35

O'Donoghue, Dr Christine, 108
Obstetric physiotherapist, 36
Obstetrician, 116
Occupational therapist(s), 27
Old age, 4
Onset of periods (menarche), 2
Operation (surgery), 67, 98, 100, 105, 107, 113, 132, 139, 140
Orthopaedic medicine, 106–7
Orthopaedic specialist, 97, 113, 140
Orthotics, 98
Ossification, 40

Osteoarthritis (osteoarthrosis, wear-and-tear degeneration), 8, 42, 133, 136
Osteochondritis, osteochondrosis, 138
Osteomalacia, 146
Osteopath, 93, 98, 102–4, 107, 123, 151
Osteopathy, 67, 81, 102–4
Osteophyte(s), 42, 136, 144
Osteoporosis (brittle bones), 80, 132, 135, 146, 147
Outer leg-bone (fibula), 60
Over-stretch, 13, 73
Overload, 13, 69, 70, 211
Overuse strains, 13, 19, 41

Paget's disease, 137, 146
Pain Clinic(s), 67, 118
Pain control, 64, 85, 89–91
Pain diary, 91
Pain pattern, 65, 83–4, 121, 125, 143
Painkillers, 67, 88, 147
Painting and decorating, 32, 92
Palmer, Mr David, 101
Palpation, 128
Parachuting, 7, 8, 9, 123, 141
Paraesthesiae ('pins and needles'), 72
Paralysis, 9, 48, 59, 85, 130, 141
Paramedical professions, 93–4, 95–104, 112
Passive Neck Flexion Test, 129
Pectoral muscles, 4, 62, 134, 213
Pelvic tilt, 4, 174
Pelvis, 1, 6, 12, 18, 26, 36, 39, 43–4, 45, 51, 53, 57, 70, 79, 101, 137
Periods (menstruation), 2, 79, 92, 202
Peripheral nerves, 48–50
Peripheral nervous system, 48
Pets, 25
Photographer, 29
Physical education teacher, 8, 87, 154
Physical examination, 94, 126–9
Physical tests, 127, 153–78
Physiotherapist(s), physical therapist(s), 27, 36, 93, 98, 99–100, 106, 108, 112, 133, 151, 184, 218

Physiotherapy, 67, 99–100, 137, 148, 152
Pillow(s), 37–8, 92
'Pins and needles' (paraesthesiae), 72
Piriformis muscle, 60
Piriformis syndrome, 137
Pistol shooting, 199
Plantar fasciitis, 146
Plaster of Paris, 104, 143
Pleurisy, 74, 149
Plyometrics, 205
Podiatrist, 98
Pool exercises (hydrotherapy), 183–4
Postural control, 1–3
Postural habits, 3, 69, 153
Postural muscles, 21
Posture, 15, 89–90, 100, 106, 119, 146
Power, 199, 207
Powerlifting, 9, 207
Pregnancy, 26, 36, 74, 82–3, 92, 102, 116, 202
Pressure sores, 17, 141
Prolapsed disc, 130
Prophylactic taping, 7
Proprioceptive neuromuscular facilitation (PNF), 110, 202
Protection, 50–1
Protective headgear, 87
Psoas major muscle, 59
Psoriatic arthritis, 146
Psychiatric treatment, 98
Psychologist, 98, 151
Psychotherapist, 98
PT Bouncers (mini-trampolines), 211
Puberty, 41
Pubic bones, 39, 44
Pubic joint, symphysis, 12, 45, 53
Pulse rate, 152

Quadratus lumborum muscle, 58
Quadriceps muscles, 5, 59, 178
Quadriplegia, 86, 141

Racket games, 4, 54, 160, 172
Radial nerve, 50
Radicular (root) pain, 71–2
'Real shortening' of one leg, 5, 140

Referred (radiating) pain, 67, 70, 83, 102, 111, 122, 125, 180
Reflexes, 128
Reflexologist(s), 98, 151
Reflexology, 67, 105
Reiters disease, 146
Relative rest, 6
Relaxation, 17, 126
Remedial (rehabilitation) exercises, 6, 16, 38, 100, 106, 115–17, 118, 119, 132, 134, 137, 138, 143, 144, 145, 147, 148, 151, 152, 154–6, 179–98
Repetitive stress, 9
Rest, 88–9, 104, 126
Resting positions, 133, 137
Resuscitation, 86
Rheumatoid arthritis, 133, 137, 146, 148–9, 180
Rheumatologist, 97, 104
Rhomboid muscles, 61
Rib(s), 1, 40, 46, 50, 51, 53, 59, 62, 71, 146
Rifle shooting, 200
Risk factors, 8–14
Rock climbing, 59
Roller skating, 87
Root (radicular) pain, 71–2
Rotational stresses, 7, 200
Rower(s), 14, 142
Rowing, 13–14, 139, 181, 200, 205
Rowing ergometer, 206, 210, 211
Rugby, 8, 12, 181, 208
Running, 12–13, 54, 60, 79, 151, 170, 200, 205

Sacralization, 42
Sacroiliac joint(s), 5, 11, 12, 26, 43, 44, 45, 46, 53, 59, 61, 70, 79, 137, 146
Sacrum, 39, 41, 43, 44, 49
Safety practices, 85
Sailing, 150
Scans, 81, 94, 147
Scapula (shoulder blade), 40, 53, 54, 59
Scheuermann's disease, S. kyphosis, 138
Schmorl's nodes, 138
Schnell exercise system, 208

School, 18
Sciatic nerve, 50, 72, 137
Sciatica, 72, 139
Sclerosing therapy, 107
Scoliosis, 3, 11, 131, 139
Sculling, 14, 54
Seat-bone (ischial tuberosity), 44, 60, 174
Second opinion, 97
Self-diagnosis, 84, 152
Self-help measures, 16, 87–8, 100, 114, 117, 118
Sensation nerves, 48
Septic arthritis, 133, 149
Serratus anterior muscle(s), 62
Sex, 36
Shearing forces, 7, 9, 13, 28, 29, 41
Shiatsu, 98, 105
Shin-bone (tibia), 60
Shingles, 150
Shock absorption, 10, 52, 170, 178
Shoes, 10, 35–6, 90, 140, 206
Shooting, 199, 200
Shop assistant, 29
Short leg syndrome, 140
Shot putting, 11
Shoulder blade (scapula), 40, 53, 54, 59
Shoulder girdle, 1, 4, 12, 19, 52, 53, 54
Shoulder(s), 4, 5, 6, 9, 21, 53, 59, 71, 170, 171, 176, 200
Show jumping, 8, 9, 85, 200
Signs and symptoms, 121
Sit-and-reach stretch, 173
Sitting, 1, 17–21, 52, 65, 89, 125
Sjorgen's syndrome, 104
Skateboarding, 87
Ski-jumping, 8
Skiing, 8, 150, 200, 205
Skin sensation, 128
Sleeping, 37, 67, 89
Sling, 6
'Slipped disc', 106
Slow-twitch muscle fibres, 2
Slump Test, 129
Sneeze, 57, 59, 65, 131
Soccer (football), 5, 12, 200
Social worker, 151
Society of Orthopaedic Medicine, 106

Somatic nervous system, 48
Somatic pain, 69–71
Spasm, 2, 6, 73, 90, 100, 105, 108, 109, 128, 135, 179
Speed, 199, 204–7
Speedboat racing, 9
Spinal column, 1, 39
Spinal cord (neuraxis, medulla spinalis), 1, 39, 48-50, 51
Spinal cord injury, 8, 48, 59, 85, 133–4, 141
Spinal joint(s), 6, 7, 44–7
Spinal nerve(s), 39, 49, 64, 71
Spinal stenosis, 113, 141
Spine, 1
Spinous processes, 41, 42, 59, 134
'Splits', 10
Spondylolisthesis (bone slippage), 142–3
Spondylolysis, 142, 143–4
Spondylosis, 136, 144
Sportesse exercise system, 208
Sports bags, 30
Sports coach, 8, 87, 109, 154, 201
Sports instructor, 8
Spotters, 212
Sprinting, 60, 208
Squash, 11, 137, 150
Squat exercise, 178, 191
Standing, 1, 21, 52, 65, 125
Static (isometric) muscle work, 55, 209
'Step class', 205
Sternum (breast-bone), 40, 51, 175
Still, Dr Andrew, 102, 108
Stoddard, Dr Alan, 108
Straight-leg-raise test, 128, 137
Strength, 9, 199, 207–18
Strengthening exercises, 185–93
Stress, 19, 61, 75, 98, 136
Stress (fatigue) fracture, 123, 142
Stretcher, 7, 86
Stretching exercises, 194–6, 202–3
Stroke, 48
Suitcases, 28
Supermarket, 29
Suppling exercises, 202
Support, 50–1

Support belt, 24, 28
Supraspinatus muscle(s), 171
Surgeon(s), 97, 106 , 113, 131, 140
Surgery (operation), 67, 98, 100, 105, 107, 113, 132, 139, 140
Sustained natural apophyseal glides (SNAGS), 110
Swimming, 54, 59, 183, 200, 208
Syndesmosis, syndesmoses, 44, 45
Symphysis pubis, 43
Synovial joint(s), 44, 148

Tae kwon do, 87
Tailbone (coccyx), 39, 41, 43, 44, 49, 107
Taping, 7
Taxi driver, 23
Teenage growth period, 4, 6, 8, 14, 41, 213
Teenager(s), 2, 24, 30, 68, 79, 124, 138, 151, 202, 203, 211
Telephone, 21
Television, 18, 19
Tendon(s), 39
Tennis, 10, 48, 79, 89, 136, 137, 139, 200
Tension tests (for the nervous system), 129
Teres major muscle(s), 59
Thoracic kyphosis, 3, 134
Throwing events, 11, 123, 160, 172, 200
Tibia (shin-bone), 60
Tinnitus, 102
Toe-touching exercise, 204
Tooth-brushing, 7
Torticollis ('wry neck', 'crick' in the neck), 144–5
Traction, 107, 111–12, 131, 132, 136, 139, 150
Traction forces, 7, 9
Trampolining, 9, 140
Tranquillizers, 67
Transcutaneous electrical nerve stimulation (TENs), 114
Transitional vertebra(e), 42
Transversospinalis muscles, 58
Trapezius muscle(s), 29, 61, 74, 136, 170

'Trapped nerve', 71, 72, 131
Treadmill(s), 205
Treatment(s), 94, 104–20
Trendelenberg's sign, 60
Triceps muscles, 5
'Trigger points', 133, 136
Triple jump, 9
Trolley(s), 29, 30
Truck driver, 23
True shortening (of the leg), 5,
    140
Tuberculosis, 149
Tumbling, 10
Tumour(s), 74

Ulcerative colitis, 146
Ulnar nerve, 50
Ultrasound, 101, 113, 114, 137
Upper Limb Tension Tests
    (ULTTs), 129

Valsalva manoeuvre, 52, 214
Van driver, 23
Vascular referred pain, 71
Vaulting, 10
Vertebra(e), 39, 41–3, 85
Vertebral artery insufficiency,
    34, 145
Vertebral body, bodies, 41, 49,
    148
Vertebral column, 1, 39, 41, 45,
    51, 58
Veterinary surgeon(s), 25
Viral infection, 61, 74, 136,
    144, 149–52
Visceral manipulation, 103
Visceral referred pain, 71
Vitamins, 79
Volleyball, 208

Walking, 5, 125, 142, 205
Warm baths, 34, 90–1
Warm-down (cool-down), 181,
    201
Warm-up, 181, 201
Washing, 33–6
Water intake, 78, 126
Wear-and-tear degeneration
    (osteoarthrosis), 8, 42, 133, 136
Wedge cushion, 20
Wedge fracture 133, 135
Wedging (of vertebral bodies),
    134

Weight training, 181, 207–18
Weightlifting, 9, 207–18
Wheelchair athletes, 12, 200
Wheelchair user, 17, 69, 141
Whiplash injury, 145–6
'Winged scapula', 62
Working environment(s), 15, 19
World Confederation for
    Physical Therapy (WCPT), 99
Wrestling, 8
'Wry neck' (torticollis, 'crick' in
    the neck), 144–5

X-rays, 42, 69, 94, 102, 106,
    122, 136, 142, 143, 147

Zygapophyseal (facet) joints,
    42, 44, 45, 49, 53, 70, 132–3,
    144